CONSULTATION, EDUCATION AND PREVENTION IN COMMUNITY MENTAL HEALTH

CONSULTATION, EDUCATION AND PREVENTION IN COMMUNITY MENTAL HEALTH

Edited by

DAVID R. RITTER, Ed.D.

Director of Consultation and Education
Rutland Mental Health Service
Rutland, Vermont

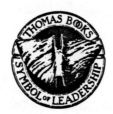

CHARLES C THOMAS • PUBLISHER

Springfield • Illinois • U.S.A.

Published and Distributed Throughout the World by

CHARLES C THOMAS • PUBLISHER
2600 South First Street
Springfield, Illinois, U.S.A. 62717

© *1982 by* CHARLES C THOMAS • PUBLISHER

ISBN 0-398-04717-0

Library of Congress Catalog Card Number: 82-5837

With THOMAS BOOKS *careful attention is given to all details of
manufacturing and design. It is the Publisher's desire to present books that
are satisfactory as to their physical qualities and artistic possibilities and
appropriate for their particular use. THOMAS BOOKS will be true to those
laws of quality that assure a good name and good will.*

Printed in the United States of America

I-R5-1

Library of Congress Cataloging in Publication Data

Main entry under title:

Consultation, education, and prevention in community
    mental health.

  Bibliography: p.
  Includes index.
  1. Community mental health services. 2. Mental ill-
ness--Prevention. 3. Mental health education. 4. Psychiatric consultation. I. Ritter, David R. [DNLM:
1. Community mental health services. 2. Referral and
consultation. 3. Health education. WM 30 C758]
RA790.C68173 1982   362.2'0425   82-5837
ISBN 0-398-04717-0   AACR2

To E.G.

CONTRIBUTORS

Anthony R. D'Augelli, Ph.D. The Pennsylvania State University, University Park, Pennsylvania

James B. Duffey, Ph.D. Montgomery County Intermediate Unit, Erdenheim, Pennsylvania

John C. Freund, Ed.D. Greater Manchester Mental Health Center, Manchester, New Hampshire

Elizabeth Girshick, Ph.D. Montgomery County Intermediate Unit, Erdenheim, Pennsylvania

Francis J. Robinson, M.Ed. Montgomery County Intermediate Unit, Erdenheim, Pennsylvania

Carolyn F. Swift, Ph.D. Southwest Community Mental Health Center, Columbus, Ohio

PREFACE

CONSULTATION and Education is, in many ways, an enigma. Despite its forte in education, C&E remains as perhaps the most misunderstood of all community mental health center services. Although possessing a capacity for the promotion of mental health, it is a service that is constantly relegated to a position secondary to that of clinical treatment. While capable of becoming self-sufficient, C&E remains financially insecure. Even though it is the program that is eminently equipped to deal with public relations and strategies of marketing, C&E itself continues to suffer from "image" problems. It is, at the very least, disquieting that such ironies exist for consultation, education and prevention, as it is a field that embodies the very intent and purpose of community mental health.

Consultation and Education is *the* service that truly seeks to promote the positive mental health of the community rather than treat individuals who become emotional casualties. The modes of consultation and education are intended to spread the wealth of knowledge possessed by mental health practitioners so that skills can be learned and information acquired by many — both caregivers and the community alike. It is the mental health service that carries the potential for broad impact, since it addresses entire systems rather than individuals. It is the arena of consultation, education and prevention programs that poses exciting opportunities for the C&E practitioner. Unfortunately, it is also a field that can lead to frustration and seemingly endless barriers to the effective delivery of preventively oriented services.

It has been encouraging to note the considerable strides that have been made by graduate training programs in preparing mental

ix

health practitioners to function as consultants, community educators or prevention specialists. However, the gap between theory and practice remains substantial. The practitioner, upon joining a mental health center, almost universally confronts a number of unexpected barriers. Organizational dynamics, political ramifications, financial concerns, federal and state regulations, issues of professional status, difficulties in systems entry, and even functioning within an environment that places little value on C&E services are but a few of the unforeseen problems that may arise. It is issues such as these that force a prompt review of one's professional functioning, a retranslation of *expected* role into *possible* accomplishments, given the reality of community mental health today.

This is a book *by* C&E practitioners *for* C&E practitioners. It addresses an array of critical issues that confront consultation, education and prevention services and, in doing so, bridges the gap between theory and reality; between philosophy and practice. The book seeks to share the skills and insights of its contributors who, themselves, are experienced consultants, community education specialists or directors of C&E programs. The knowledge contained herein should prove valuable to the student and the C&E professional alike and, it is hoped, will serve to revitalize interest and energies in the C&E field. At the very least, the book will provide the reader with an "inside" view of the day-to-day operations, problems and potentials of community mental health consultation and education as they exist today and might exist in the future.

The book's initial chapter, authored by Anthony D'Augelli of the Pennsylvania State University, provides an introduction to and historical synthesis of mental health consultation, education and prevention. Dr. D'Augelli provides a review of the theoretical and philosophical constructs that underlie C&E as well as a number of useful typologies of the service delivery system. Superimposed upon the frameworks is his critical analysis of the field. Together, they form a solid conceptual base from which the remainder of the chapters proceed.

Chapter 2 discusses a number of program models and organizational structures that are presently used by community mental health consultation and education programs. The relative advantages and limitations of each organizational model are addressed, as is the critical role of the C&E director. The reader may find the description of an Integrated Community Service to be particularly intriguing, perhaps even controversial, as the concept strikes at the very heart of C&E as a distinct unit.

John Freund, the Director of Consultation and Education with the Aroostock (Maine) Community Mental Health Center at the time of preparation of this book, and now with the Greater Manchester Mental Health Center (New Hampshire), deals with the matter of preparing and training clinicians to function as effective consultants. Dr. Freund provides valuable insight into the personal issues, internal factors, and external conflicts that can and do arise between clinical theory and community consultation practice. Chapter 3 goes on to examine the multidisciplinary nature of C&E staffing patterns, the varying roles played by paraprofessionals, and the importance of effective use of community resources.

Chapter 4 deals with dollars and cents, the topic being the financing of Consultation and Education. Historically, C&E has paid little attention to the need for financial self-sufficiency. Recent developments on a national level have vaulted the issue of finances to the fore, making it a topic that C&E can no longer ignore.

James Duffey, Elizabeth Girshick and Francis Robinson, colleagues with the Montgomery County Intermediate Unit (Pennsylvania), collaborate on Chapter 5, on the process of consultation. Their writing is refreshing, as instead of providing the reader with the usual description of consultation methods, they delve into the subtleties of credibility, power, entry, negotiations and conflict of interest, the truely significant factors that either make or break an effective consultative relationship.

Chapter 6, on methods of evaluating consultation, education and prevention services is direct and informative. The reader will find that many of the traditional experimental and quasi-experimental designs commonly used in research are translated into practical application for C&E programs. Other evaluative methodologies, such as goal attainment scaling and performance contracting, are also discussed. A topology of levels of evaluative information is offered to assist in the planning and implementation of program evaluation. A prospective look toward the relationship of evaluation and services is attempted in keeping with C&E's entry into an era of heightened accountability.

Carolyn Swift, the Director of Prevention Programs for the Southwest Community Mental Health/Mental Retardation Center (Ohio), shares her practical experience and National perspective on the role of preventive services in community mental health. In Chapter 7, Dr. Swift provides the reader with a definitive statement on the state of the art of prevention, as it has been, and as it is likely to be for the next decade, given the economic tenor of the times. New directions in prevention services are addressed with emphasis on the preventive potentials of television as a mass media vehicle for spreading the word about positive mental health practices.

Chapter 8 concludes with a prospective look toward C&E's future, linking the challenges of the present with the opportunities of the years to come. The overriding theme of the chapter is that of integration, for the book itself and the field of C&E. It is the grassroots of C&E, its own practitioners, who possess the capacity to meet and resolve the difficult issues that lie before them and, in doing so, to revitalize C&E.

DAVID R. RITTER

CONTENTS

CONSULTATION, EDUCATION
AND PREVENTION IN
COMMUNITY MENTAL HEALTH

Chapter 1

HISTORICAL SYNTHESIS
OF CONSULTATION AND EDUCATION

ANTHONY R. D'AUGELLI

"Typhus was conquered when the doctors discovered the part played by the louse in transmitting it. Where is the Louse in Mental Health?" (Comment of an anonymous participant at the 1958 National Assembly on Mental Health Education).

WHAT do the following events have in common: a brochure advertising a community mental health center, a monthly meeting of an interagency organization, a curriculum to teach skills to child care workers, a television program on stress, after school activities for troubled high school students, a course on human relations for middle management of business and industry, a newspaper column on how to cope with life events, and a "warm line" for confused parents? What do these people have in common: an indigenous worker discussing learning disabilities with inner-city parents, a social worker talking with an elderly woman conducting a program for the recently widowed, a psychologist

The author would like to thank those colleagues who commented on an earlier draft on this chapter: Lewis Katoff, Anthony Broskowski, Robert Ehrlich, Steven Danish, Thomas Brandon, David Snow, Richard Marold, Richard Munger, Robert Hess, Roger Williams, Betty Tableman and Ferdinand Hassler. I would also like to thank the many C&E directors and staff members with whom I met. This chapter was completed during a sabbatical leave granted by the College of Human Development at The Pennsylvania State University.

consulting with an organization, and a psychiatrist discussing the topic of depression with the host of a local talk show? The common denominator is C&E — Consultation and Education — one of the essential services provided to communities by community mental health centers (CMHCs). The first set of events described above are activities that could be provided by C&E programs; the second set are examples of the kind of people who comprise a C&E staff.

C&E is a specific category of mental health service that federally funded CMHCs must offer. C&E stands in distinction from other mandated services in its focus on maximizing the impact of mental health services in communities. Services designed to extend mental health resources to community caregivers (consultation) and services to inform the general public about mental health (education) are "nonclinical" in nature. In addition, C&E units in CMHCs are distinctly capable of grappling with the need to develop prevention programs toward a goal of decreasing the number of incidents of disorder in the community. A service modality that is intrinsically aimed at increasing the "spread of effect" of mental health service has much to offer in the effort to deal with both the current prevalence and the future prevention of psychosocial stress.

Despite the unique nature of this kind of mental health service, C&E programs are constantly troubled by confusion of goals. Clearly, C&E is a nonclinical service, but it is often easier to describe what C&E is *not* than to describe what it *is*. Since C&E is such a broad conceptual umbrella, definitional problems are persistent. The role of consultation, education and prevention within each CMHC is defined by that particular context. In some centers, C&E units engage mostly in case finding, case consultation and publicity. In other centers, programs stress prevention activities rather than support of clinical services, considering the latter as an inappropriate C&E task. The nature and number of staff across different C&E units varies tremendously as does the perceived support and security of C&E personnel. While some C&E programs are carefully integrated into the CMHC, others are "gypsy units"[1] whose purpose and activities are poorly understood by

[1] As much as I would like to claim ownership to this label, honesty impels me to give credit to Lois Brozenak, Beaver County (PA) MH/MR Program.

other CMHC staff. C&E services are essential to the survival of community mental health, yet C&E is currently poorly defined, operationalized in very idiosyncratic ways, and seldom adequately evaluated. It appears that C&E units share little except a federal mandate.

This chapter will review the role of Consultation and Education in community mental health centers and will provide a critical overview. A brief history of C&E services will be provided, the current status of consultation and mental health education will be reviewed, current problems of definition will be discussed, and the relationship of C&E to prevention will be described. Issues related to fiscal problems, conceptual frameworks, the development of a C&E knowledge base, professional preparation for C&E and evaluation issues will also be presented. Finally, future directions will be suggested.

Throughout this analysis, the critical question of the relationship of C&E to primary prevention will be highlighted. The concept of primary prevention leads to a redesign of mental health services toward the provision of psychosocial assets to communities, families and individuals. For mental health, the main institutional settings for the struggle to energize resources for primary prevention are C&E units. To the extent that C&E programs succeed, so too will primary prevention. If C&E falters under the considerable definitional, organizational, and fiscal strains that presently exist, so too will primary prevention remain but an ideal beyond reach. Mental health services may slowly retreat from primary prevention and return to an emphasis on treatment unless C&E practitioners can clarify the role of C&E in prevention. It is no exaggeration to state that the future of C&E in CMHCs is quite uncertain. The challenge of the future will be whether or not C&E can overcome its current marginality as a mental health specialty and become a viable force for the promotion of mental health in communities.

HISTORICAL BACKGROUND

The history of Consultation and Education reflects the transition of mental health services from institutional to community-based care provided through CMHCs. As a service modality, C&E

provided a concrete approach to address major problems in the delivery of mental health services that were identified in the early 1960s. Four major problem areas were (and are) salient in the evolution of community mental health. First, despite considerable advances in the technology of remedial behavior change, the effectiveness of routine psychotherapeutic care remained, at best, modest. Second, epidemiological data on the prevalence of psychological problems consistently identified more individuals and families than were currently service recipients or than could possibly receive adequate care. Third, a consensus emerged that future mental health intervention must consider environmental, ecological and community influences on psychosocial stress. Fourth, current practice provided an uneven distribution of mental health resources in terms of geographical maldistributions (rural areas and inner cities are notoriously underserved), as well as age-related (the young and the old receive fewer services) and minority status-related inequities. Research evidence also pointed to a new direction for future mental health services:

> Research grants made available by NIMH after 1957 and by other sources to demonstrate improved treatment methods showed that alternatives to hospitalization are possible and effective; that emergency care and crisis intervention avert longer hospitalization and are effective in restoring functioning; that rehabilitation programs do help restore mentally handicapped persons through sheltered living and working arrangements; that follow-up services decrease readmissions; *that consultation to community agencies can be useful;* that paraprofessionals of various kinds perform useful psychotherapeutic and other functions in appropriate settings; that administrative and treatment information systems are possible to install and use for program planning; and that the availability of adequate community services decreases state hospital admissions. (Yolles, 1977, pp. 25-26; emphasis added)

The "bold new approach" of community mental health was viewed as a solution to these difficult problems, and a system of community mental health centers became the institutional consequence. Within these centers, a service that intrinsically embodied a "multiplier effect," one that was designed to be influential with larger numbers of recipients, seemed to hold much promise. Indeed, it was logical to assume that services which emphasized prevention and mental health promotion would be prominent in CMHCs.

C&E was included as one of five services required for a CMHC to receive funding under the Community Mental Health Systems Act of 1963 (Public Law 88-164). Although not defined in detail,[2] C&E's unusual role was clear to its early supporters in NIMH. As an avenue for prevention, C&E was viewed as a cost-effective way of improving service delivery. Stanley Yolles, then NIMH director, wrote as follows in 1966:

> Consultation and education is a promising new mental health tool. . . .
> Four of the five essential elements of service required of a comprehensive community mental health center focus on new methods of treatment and care. The fifth, consultation and education to community agencies and professionals, is concerned with the prevention of mental illness and the promotion of mental health. (Quoted in Howery, Note 1, p. 1)

This conception of C&E focused on community *agencies* and *caregivers* (professionals) as the prime target of C&E endeavors. C&E personnel were expected to work with social welfare agencies, prisons, schools, and other relevant institutions having direct contact with clients with mental health problems. The focus on consultation to other human service agencies can clearly be seen in a later definition that Yolles provided:

> The rationale for the national mental health program also included (as an essential service) the establishment of a consultation and education service, known as C&E. C&E was designed to achieve several things. It was seen first as a means to develop preventive mental health services in a community by requiring the CMHC staffs to initiate community-wide exchange on a routine basis with the staffs of all relevant community agencies. In so doing, it would operate to break down professional isolation and agency barriers to the benefit of the staffs, the clients and the taxpayers. (Yolles, 1977, p. 40)

Consultation and education were not conceived as two discrete functions but rather as a generic service that was "indirect"[3] in its

---

[2]The only actual mention of C&E occurs in the Regulations for Title II of P.L. 88-164. Section 54.212 defines five essential services: inpatient services, outpatient services, partial hospitalization services, emergency services, and C&E. C&E services are "services available to community agencies and professional personnel."

[3]The Council on Prevention of the National Council of Community Mental Health Centers has successfully lobbied to stop the use by NIMH and others of the term "indirect services" to describe C&E. The argument is that these services are often quite "direct." Most mental health education, for example, is a direct transmission to a group of recipients. The term "indirect" may have gathered too many surplus meanings (including "less important") to capture accurately C&E services.

impact on individuals and their families. C&E, as it was practiced at this point, consisted of case consultation in which an expert from the CMHC would visit another human service agency that was troubled by a specific client. The concept of prevention was used in its broadest sense. Certainly primary prevention was seldom practiced.

C&E thus began its institutional history as a poorly defined set of "indirect" services linking the CMHC with other human services. In practice, C&E provided support to CMHC clinical services by case finding, case consultation, training of center personnel in new treatment methods, public relations about the center, and the development of informational campaigns, usually about mental illnesses. The unique contribution of C&E for prevention was lost in the process. As Perlmutter and Silverman (1973) remark;

> Consultation was defined as a problem-solving service with emphasis on "relaying help to the person in need"; education was defined as its knowledge-building twin, designed to help citizens maintain their well-being through more knowledge and new behavior patterns resulting from this knowledge. . . . In reality the prevention objective remained an ideal and was not implemented in practice; the major focus around the nation was on treatment services. (Pp. 116-117)

The ambiguity of C&E in the 1963 CMHC legislation improved somewhat in subsequent amendments to the Community Mental Health Center Act. In the 1975 ammendments (Public Law 94-63), C&E activities were specifically described as services that

(i) are for a wide range of individuals and entities, including health professionals, schools, courts, state and local law enforcement and correctional agencies, members of the clergy, public welfare agencies, health service delivery agencies, and other appropriate entities; and

(ii) include a wide range of activities (other than the provision of direct clinical services) designed to: (1) develop effective mental health programs in the center's catchment area; (2) promote the coordination of the provision of mental health services among various entities serving the center's catchment area; (3) increase the awareness of residents of the center's catchment area of the nature of mental health problems and the types of mental health services available; and (4) promote the prevention and control of rape and the proper treatment of the victims of rape.

These amendments also include a significant institutional method to force CMHCs to give C&E prominence. Congress provided specific funding for C&E as one of twelve mandated services,[4] giving C&E at least a fiduciary life of its own. One year after the 1975 amendments were passed, Stanley Yolles made this optimistic prognosis at a conference on community psychiatry:

> C&E has not developed as effectively as had been planned. The idea was new; in fact, this was the first time in any federal health statute where a preventive service has been declared to be mandatory. In the 1975 amendments, provision is made to provide for a system of grants, specifically available to C&E programs in CMHC's. . . .The dollar incentive should stimulate the preventive aspects of the entire CMHC program. (Yolles, 1977, p. 41)

CURRENT STATUS

Whereas the legislative history of C&E is comparatively easy to reconstruct, the actual nature of C&E activities in local communities is impossible to document. The few empirical studies that exist are limited to small samples of C&E programs. In an impressionistic study of four CMHCs in Philadelphia, Perlmutter and Silverman (1973) found only one center with a clearly elaborated philosophy of C&E. C&E programs appeared to dichotomize into those focused on prevention through community organization and those oriented toward supporting treatment efforts. Perlmutter (1974) later argued that C&E prevention activities were always likely to be in jeopardy within the medically oriented CMHC structure. A study of ten CMHCs in the Midwest (Mazade, 1974) found a relationship between C&E practice and CMHC organizational structure. Those centers rated more flexible in their structure encouraged program-oriented consultation, while consultations from CMHCs in general hospitals were more likely to be case oriented. A study by Miller, Mazade and Muller (1978), although not directly querying C&E activities, found that 173 mental health centers reported that 63.3 percent of their staff hours were de-

---

[4]The other eleven services are inpatient services, outpatient services, partial hospitalization, emergency services, screening services, follow-up services, transitional housing arrangements, children's services, services for the elderly, alcoholism services and drug abuse services.

voted to treatment services with the remainder focused on services "considered proactive and focused on social network support, preventive services, mental health education, and services in response to difficulties encountered during normal development and growth" (p. 192). To date, the most useful information about C&E services comes from an intensive study conducted by Bader and Ketterer for the Michigan Department of Mental Health (Note 2). Focusing on four CMHCs in Wayne County, Michigan, this study used archival records of CMHCs, interviews with program staff, field observations and case study methods to discover issues in the delivery of C&E services. Bader and Ketterer found that 82.3 percent of C&E programs' goals focused on services to individuals and the community, 4.2 percent of their goals were related to the CMHC and 13.5 percent were C&E maintenance and survival goals. The three most frequently cited community services were mental health education, caregiver consultation and training and network/coalition building. They suggest that much work is needed in clarifying the role of C&E in CMHCs, in delineating the goals of C&E services, in describing roles, skills, and training, in managing C&E, and in developing information and evaluation systems for C&E services. The thoroughness of the Bader and Ketterer study makes it a reference point for any future national analysis of C&E.

The only national data on C&E are available through the Division of Biometry of NIMH. This information, collected annually using the Inventory of Comprehensive Community Mental Health Centers, focuses on the number of staff hours spent during a selected month on consultation (subdivided into case-oriented, staff development and/or continued education, and program oriented) and public information. Consultation services to center staff are explicitly excluded. The Division of Biometry accumulates this data and prepares a report each year. Based on these reports, called Provisional Data on Federally Funded Community Mental Health Centers (NIMH, Note 3), Hassler (Note 4) has developed this composite picture of federally supported C&E services up to 1977:

1. Children are by far the main recipients of C&E services.
2. Less than 5 percent of the total staff time of the centers was devoted to C&E.

3. A minor increase has occurred in the amount of C&E services devoted to older adults.
4. Most C&E staff have at least a bachelor's degree.
5. The percentage of total CMHC staff hours for C&E has progressively diminished since the early 1970s.
6. Considerable variability exists on nearly all indices of C&E activity, including amount of staff time, outside funding generated by the C&E unit and focus of the program activities.

Table 1-I summarizes the percentage of staff time devoted to the different kinds of recipient groups.

Table 1-I

DISTRIBUTION OF C&E STAFF TIME (%) BY RECIPIENT TYPE

Recipient	1973	1974	1975	1976	1977	1978
Children	40.4*	38.7*	45.8	42.4	37.2	32.4
General Public	NA	NA	2.9	3.0	12.5	15.0
State and Local Law	11.7	8.1	9.4	9.1	8.3	7.4
Health Services	9.9	8.9	8.6	9.5	7.9	8.6
Substance Abuse	7.2	8.7	5.8	7.9	6.8	5.8
Other Mental Health	6.8	7.1	7.5	8.4	6.7	6.8
Public Welfare	12.1	8.6	6.6	6.7	5.8	4.4
Elderly	3.3	4.0	4.2	4.9	5.7	6.7
Other	8.6	15.9	9.2	9.1	9.1	12.9

*School Consultation only.

From F. Hassler, Overview of the national C&E data, unpublished report available from F. Hassler, Staff College — NIMH, 5635 Fishers Lane, Rockville, MD, 20852; also from National Institute of Mental Health, provisional data on federally funded community mental health centers, 1977-1978.

The current status of C&E services, thus, can only be the subject of informed speculation. The NIMH data presented above show the modest levels of funding allocated to C&E units within CMHCs. Whether or not a decreasing trend is fact (a consequence of centers "graduating" from their staffing grants) or artifact is unknown, although Swift (1980) has argued that these data conservatively estimate actual C&E activities. Despite the vicissitudes of funding, a more fundamental problem exists for consultation and education, the problem of domain. Federal support has not resulted in a distinct set of C&E services that must be provided to local communities. Klein writes (Note 5):

> Judging by the apparent variations, a mental health center's C&E program *is* what a C&E program *does*, and the latter reflects considerable variance from center to center depending on the background and skills of the C&E staff, the predilections of those responsible for managing the CMHC, the felt needs of influential community groups and institutions, and the like. There is no generally agreed upon model of the C&E worker, let alone of a C&E program. (P. 1)

Whether this diversity of C&E activities from center to center reflects a healthy sensitivity to community context and needs or is simply conceptual chaos[5] is perhaps less important than the larger national consequences of the patchwork nature of current C&E activities. Many C&E programs flounder due to uncertain direction and purpose, having little sense of what problems need to be emphasized as priorities. Since the possibilities are endless — everything from an informal chat with a chief of police, to developing a media campaign on parenting, to helping a local industry redesign its ecology, to conducting groups for midlife career change can legitimately be justified as a C&E activity — a systematic process of planning is required. The vulnerability of C&E activities to larger institutional pressures makes the construction of distinct C&E goals even more problematic. A number of C&E staff provide services that cannot be appropriately considered as C&E but that are politically necessary with the CMHC and help "keep the peace." As Snow and Swift[6] have recently remarked;

---

[5]Yolles (1977) discusses the conflict between CMHC advocates of two opposing views: those who call for an exclusive focus on services for those already mentally ill and those who argue for an emphasis on righting social and economic problems. He suggests that this is a local issue: "If one looks dispassionately at the regulations and guidelines, it is obvious that each community mental health center, each state, and each city or county has a great opportunity to make of each program what they will — based on a consensus of the perceived needs of each catchment area" (p. 42).

[6]Snow, D.L., and Swift, C. *Consultation and education: Definition and philosophy.* Available from D.L. Snow, Department of Psychiatry, Yale University, 34 Park Street, New Haven, Connecticut 06519.

We feel that some of the activities in which C&E staff are asked to engage within the larger CMHC involve an inappropriate use of C&E time. Resources designated for C&E are often diverted into clinical services, or staff are utilized to carry out central administrative functions or to serve in a community liaison or public relations role. (P. 7)

Since there is so little clarity about what C&E is, there is little chance for a constituency to develop support for C&E services. The result is that fiscal and other resources are drained to treatment services (which have gained powerful lobbies in most communities), and C&E is slowly transformed from a prevention service to an adjunct that supports treatment. Thus, the visibility of a C&E as an activity for which increased expenditure is essential has not been achieved. As Maclennan writes (1979),

If there are declining funds for staffing, and reimbursements for direct services are on a fee-for-service basis, it is inevitable that primary emphasis will be placed on treating patients even though this may be, in the long run, more expensive. (P. 94)

Despite the many problems, there remains a basic commitment to the perspective embodied by C&E services. The perspective has been described by Ketterer and Bader (Note 2) as involving the following:

1. A commitment to citizen involvement in CMHC activities
2. A commitment to the development of community resources and social supports
3. A commitment to prevention
4. A commitment to an explanatory model of human behavior that views problems as a function of the external environment as well as of deficits in individual coping skills
5. A commitment to a "seeking" or active mode of service delivery in contrast to a "waiting" mode of rehabilitative services

Such an ideology is consistent, of course, with community mental health in general. In addition to holding these views, C&E workers have another general commonality, that being the use of two sets of problem-solving strategies that disseminate mental health resources in economical yet powerful ways — consultation to community caregivers and systems, and education of the community at large about and for mental health. These two mental health technologies will each be reviewed briefly.

MENTAL HEALTH CONSULTATION

The recognition that professional manpower resources within community mental health were inadequate to meet the demand for services led to several innovative developments. One of these developments was mental health consultation. In medical circles, the most typical consultation occurs between one expert physician (the consultant) and another physician (the consultee) whose patient's care is at issue. In mental health consultation, however, the consultant typically works with someone who is *not* a mental health specialist. Indeed, this distinction marks the unique focus of mental health consultation. Mental health consultation developed on the premise that others in the community are involved in mental health, that these others (usually called gatekeepers) could benefit from interaction with a mental health professional, and that this process, over time, could have a more powerful impact than traditional psychotherapeutic services, which could be delivered only to a small percentage of those in need. As Caplan (1972) writes,

> Many mental health clinicians regard consultation to clergy and other caregivers, such as public-health nurses, general practitioners, teachers, and the police as the pivot of their own community work. . . . Since there are far too few clinicians to accomplish this task alone, they must mobilize the efforts of other caregivers by convincing them that while they are doing their own jobs, they can also help mental health personnel to do theirs. (P. 38)

Mental health consultation has a long history (see Levine & Levine, 1970; Meyers, Parsons & Martin, 1979), but it was not until Caplan's work (1964, 1970) that it was carefully conceptualized. The definition remains apt.

> By the term "mental health consultation," I designate the use of this method as part of a community program for the promotion of mental health and for the prevention, treatment, and rehabilitation of mental disorder. Much, if not most, of the work with actual or potential patients in such programs is currently being carried out by professional workers who have no specialized training in psychiatry, psychology, or psychiatric social work, namely, nurses, teachers, family doctors, pediatricians, clergyman, probation officers, policeman, welfare workers, and so forth. Recruitment and training possibilities in the mental health professions are such that this state of affairs is likely to continue indefinitely. It seems important, therefore, that a significant proportion of

the time and energies of mental health specialists be focused on improving the operations of these other caregiving professionals in relation to
mental health and mental disorder. (Caplan, 1964, p. 213)

There is little doubt that Caplan's pioneering view, along with
those of Erich Lindemann (1944) and Irving Berlin (1954, 1964,
1977), helped to popularize mental health consultation and influenced the inclusion of C&E in CMHC legislation. Caplan includes the explicit recognition that consultation and education are
interwoven processes for prevention:

Consultees learn how to pull themselves up by their bootstraps. The
goal of consultation is not just to help the consultee with a particular
case. The real focus of consultation is help plus education. (Caplan,
1977, p. 18)

Thus, consultation is not merely a dispensation of expert advice about a specific problem but is focused on the consultee as an
influence on many community residents. The consultee's organizational role is central to mental health consultation, and it is
through effecting change in community institutions and social
systems that a widespread preventive impact is achieved. Placing
consultation firmly within a community mental health ideology,
Hassol and Cooper (1970) state:

The involvement is with the institutions of the community and the
major responsibility is toward populations, including not only those
seeking direct clinical services, but also those unable or unwilling to use
such services and those not in need of them. Consultation, therefore, is
not an attempt to make wholesale what were previously retail psychiatric services. Rather, the consultation approach seeks access to populations and to the social and emotional environments in which people live
for purposes of facilitating emotionally sound psychological growth in
as many people as possible. (P. 704).

The radiating effect of consultation is its main power, but the
approach can be applied in very different ways. Kelly (1970), in
an excellent description of models for preventive interventions,
presents three consultation strategies: (1) the *clinical approach*
toward individuals or small groups, e.g. a teacher or a group of
school nurses; (2) the *organizational approach* in which the behavior of people in organizational systems is the focus, e.g. a neighborhood, a factory, a prison; and (3) the *community development*
approach, which seeks to create opportunities for communities to
change and guide the planned future of the collectivity. A similar
categorization of general goals of consultation is provided by

Cherniss (1976), who distinguishes four areas: (1) organizational structure and process; (2) the mental health of individuals; (3) group or organizational environment; and (4) technology dissemination. Consultation as a professional activity is a dissemination of mental health resources, but the target of the consultation may vary considerably. The range of consultation activities is well described by Plog and Ahmed (1977):

> The mental health consultant may be called upon to diagnose the meaning of the behaviors of an individual (client), delicately handle the emotional problems of a consultee, defuse a potentially explosive political situation threatening to destroy a community organization, work constructively in a small-group setting, help plan the mental health programs and services for his consultee agency, and work effectively with a broad spectrum of ages, income groups, and ethnic backgrounds — all within a single day. (P. 4)

Nearly every conceivable consultee has been involved in mental health consultation. In its most recent listing of consultation recipients, NIMH (Note 6) lists these eleven:

1. State and local law enforcement and correctional agencies
2. Facilities and organizations concerned with alcoholism
3. Facilities and organizations concerned with other drug abuse
4. Facilities and organizations concerned with family planning
5. Mental health facilities not affiliated with the center
6. Health service delivery systems
7. Public welfare organizations
8. Programs and organizations for the aged
9. Facilities and organizations concerned with children other than school
10. General public and organizations not listed above
11. Public and private primary and secondary schools, colleges, and universities

Many of these organizations are formal human service agencies. The list does not explicitly include work with clergy, industry, self-help groups, community groups, or informal helpers. Therefore, NIMH's listing of consultees unfortunately leads to an underestimation of the amount of consultation provided to gatekeepers and others who do not have a formal human service role. A recent critique of these definitions by the Southern Regional Education Board (SREB, Note 7) recommends a number of additional recipients:

12. Churches and church-related organizations
13. Business and industry and employment-related organizations
14. Governmental policy makers
15. Self-help and mutual support groups
16. Community and neighborhood agencies

The recognition of the power of these less formal mental health resources has led to considerable interest in the development of supportive consultative relationships between mental health centers and self-help groups, mutual support groups, and informal helpers (Caplan & Killilea, 1976; Collins & Pancoast, 1976; Gartner & Reissman, 1977; Silverman, 1978). The range of consultation has widened to go beyond those in human services. Definitions of all sixteen recipients of consultation may be found in Appendix A.

In addition to a wide range of consultees, consultation itself is of differing types. Caplan (1970) distinguished four consultation approaches: (1) client-centered case consultation in which the consultant deals with a specific case; (2) program-centered administrative consultation, which has a focus on the problems of administering a human service program; (3) consultee-centered case consultation on the work problems of the consultee that result from a lack of knowledge, skill or objectivity; and (4) consultee-centered administrative consultation in which the consultee's difficulties with programs are discussed. Heller and Monahan (1977) divide consultation activities into three areas based upon conceptual views of behavior change: (1) psychodynamic (Caplan's is placed here), (2) behavioral and (3) organizational. The focus can be on the client, the consultee or the program (or policy). Dworkin and Dworkin (1975) present four consultation models: consultee-centered, group process, social action and ecological. From a different perspective, that of consultant style, Reinking, Livesay and Kohl (1978) distinguish three types: *expert,* in which the consultant assumes that the consultee lacks the competence to solve the problem and actively suggests remedies; *resource,* where the consultant supplies knowledge that the consultee needs and leaves the decision about solutions to the consultee; and *process* through which the consultant fosters the development or problem-solving skills of the consultee and encourages and supports these efforts.

Since NIMH directives help to shape C&E activities, NIMH definitions of types of consultation are worth detailing. The annual CMHC inventory identifies three areas: case-oriented consultation, staff development and/or continued education and *agency-centered* program consultation and *community-centered* program consultation. The most recent set of definitions (NIMH, Note 6) includes two major dimensions — problem-oriented consultation and planning and development-oriented consultation. Problem-oriented consultation is further subdivided into case, staff and program consultations. Since it is likely that these newer definitions will be used in the future, they are provided in Appendix B.

The wide scope of mental health consultation makes it difficult to draw conclusions about the frequency of different kinds of consultation. NIMH data, however, are useful in demonstrating that the most typical consultation is case consultation. In 1978, CMHCs reported (NIMH, Note 8) that 40.5 percent of all consultation hours were case oriented. Staff development/continued education accounted for 24.27 percent of staff hours, and program-oriented consultation involved 35.64 percent. About one-third of the case consultations occurred in schools, and an additional 5.8 percent were in facilities that are concerned with children. Despite the stereotype that consultants work mostly to upgrade caregivers, only one-quarter of the total consultation hours were devoted to education and training. The umbrella category, program-oriented, is more easily understood by what it excludes than by what really transpires. For example, 14.4 percent of this time was devoted to the general public, but this could mean a variety of transactions ranging from a consultation with an agency administration to a training program for local advisory board members. From a different data base (19 C&E staff members in Michigan) Ketterer and Bader (Note 2) found 95 percent of staff surveyed provided caregiver consultation and training, 84 percent were involved in program and administrative consultation, and 74 percent worked toward network/coalition building and grassroots consultation. Interestingly, only 53 percent of surveyed staff reported doing case consultation. Of course, these sets of data are not directly comparable: NIMH asks *how much time* was spent; whereas Ketterer and Bader asked *whether or not* staff engaged in specific activities.

The high percentage of CMHC staff time devoted to case consultation raises the issue of the relative focus of C&E programs on preventive activities versus rehabilitative services. With a focus on identifiable clients or client "units," case consultation cannot be seen as primary prevention, although it is conceivable that these activities would be secondarily preventive in situations in which a consultee suspects possible problems. It is more likely, however, that the majority of these cases are treatment related. Pressures on the CMHC for consultation are for resolution of mental health problems of individuals. Few consultants are asked initially to modify a consultee's agency or the agency's policies so as to reduce psychiatric problems. Hassol and Cooper (1970) write:

> To people who are interested in getting some outside expert to cure or straighten out a particular individual who is of concern to the caretaking group, and without a period of interaction during which a sense of trust and collaboration can develop, the offer of consultation focused on improving the mental health problem solving of the organization sounds somewhat hollow and indeed irrelevant. (P. 708)

Whether the emphasis on case-related consultation is reasonable for C&E, or a compromising of the essential prevention mandate, is a controversial topic. A decade ago, Signell and Scott (1971) succinctly stated the issue. They commented:

> The target population (for consultation) was the sick ones. This was the same target that outpatient and inpatient services had. Consultation, then, extended responsibility not so much to a wider population, but to a wider range of caregivers. Sometimes this meant a chance for early detection, too. . . . However, from the beginning, the explicit hope was for primary prevention. . . . There was wishful thinking that consultation might affect broad social problems — sources of stress for the population and its systems. (P. 289)

The expectation that social change and community development be directed by CMHC's consultation activities may well have been an unrealistic idea. Snow and Newton's (1976) analysis of the primary tasks of CMHCs would certainly suggest that centers were unlikely to have become the focal point for preventively oriented community change. From another perspective, a more conservative yet socially useful function can be served by consultations that do not have direct primary preventive intents. This view, more appropriate in the current *zeitgeist,* is stated by Mannino and Shore (1979):

In consultations around areas that are not specifically primary prevention, such as treatment or social support programs for the severely mentally ill, elements of primary prevention are often present. For example, providing consultation to nonclinical community groups such as employer organizations, landlords, housing officials, neighborhood associations, police, and storekeepers aimed at eliciting their help in establishing socially supportive systems for the mentally ill in the community is preventive in that it raises the level of awareness and sensitivity in the community to mental health issues. Consultation thereby enables the community to function in a more humane way with all persons with problems and elevates its sense of competence and well-being through its ability to solve its own problems and plan for its own development. (P. 110)

Regardless of its focus, the technology of mental health consultation has become well-established. Several excellent models of the consultation process are available (e.g. Goodstein, 1978; Kadushin, 1977; Meyers, Parsons & Martin, 1978), as are examples of how consultation fails (e.g. Cherniss, 1977; Lepkin, 1975; Reppucci, Sarata, Saunders, McArthur & Michlin, 1973). A considerable body of research evidence to support the relevance of consultation has been well summarized by Mannino and Shore (1975) and Grady, Gibson and Trickett (1981). Furthermore, advances have occurred in delineating needs for future evaluations of consultation (e.g. Jerrel & Schulberg, 1981), especially the need to document both the process and the outcome of consultative activities. The pressure to evaluate will likely produce new developments in consultation practice. Indeed, without such pressure, consultation will likely remain an idiosyncratic process whose success (like that of psychotherapy) may be less dependent on technology transfer than on the interpersonal qualities of the consultant.

MENTAL HEALTH EDUCATION

Mental health education is a process by which factual information about some aspect of mental health is disseminated. A mental health center might, for example, offer specialized seminars in new approaches to psychotherapy for mental health professionals as well as courses for police officers on how to recognize mental problems. Virtually any topic related to the psychological well-being of the citizens of a community could be the subject of a mental health education program. (Heck, Gomez, & Adams, 1973)

This definition illuminates the scope of educational efforts for mental health. For example, during the Spring of 1980, one C&E unit in Pennsylvania offered the following educational programs to its community: Introduction to Couples' Communication, Getting Started with Personal Growth, Baby Massage Workshop, Parenting Skills with Preschoolers, Developing Confidence, Assertiveness Training, Relaxation and Stress Control, You and Your Aging Parent, Staying Psychologically Fit, How to Live on a Limited Income, Helping Yourself through Yoga, and Stress Management and Burnout Prevention for Helping Professionals. This program also distributes a parent education course, "Pierre the Pelican," to any parent with a newborn. In another center, the C&E unit distributes at the local library bookmarks that list "Tips for Tension," while in a third center a C&E staff members writes a newspaper column about life events and their stresses. All of these, and many additional activities, fall under the educational component of C&E. For many years, education was oriented toward publicizing the CMHC in the community. Any intraorganizational event that was educative in nature was provided by C&E, the most popular being in-service training. More recently, educational efforts aimed at specific target groups such as parents, the newly married, and the elderly have become the staple of the educational role of C&E. Indeed, parenting workshops and stress management workshops are ubiquitous "standard fare" in CMHCs. Because of the popularity of such programs, mental health education has become one of the most visible activities of the CMHC.

Regrettably, mental health education does not have a clear history. Perhaps the most important landmark was the 1958 National Assembly on Mental Health Education held at Cornell University. Cosponsored by the National Association for Mental Health, the American Psychiatric Association, and Pennsylvania Mental Health, Inc., this gathering of distinguishing mental health professionals explored ways to develop educational programs. Several key questions were to be addressed:

1. Can we agree on a definition of mental health?
2. Toward what goals should mental health education be directed?
3. What principles of mental health have enough support in scientific findings and clinical experience to support a mental health educational program built on them?

4. Given the objectives agreed upon and the principles identified, are there certain preferred educational techniques?

That none of these questions were adequately answered is quickly seen in the conference proceedings (National Assembly on Mental Health Education, 1960). Discussion apparently became quite heated, with major camps forming either to argue for programs that emphasized the distribution of information on mental illness or to champion efforts for and about mental health. Strong feeling was voiced about defining mental health as anything except the absence of mental illness since, by this argument, specification of components of mental health was moralizing. Agreement occurred on these general "facts of life" about mental illness:

> . . .that some mental illnesses are controllable with early and effective treatment; that there is or should be no disgrace about being or having been mentally ill; that a recovered patient might be ready to take his full share in the work and life of the community; that somehow treatment of mental illness is difficult and recovery slow. (NAMHE, 1960, p.4)

Elaine Cumming, whose own mental health education effort was an admitted dismal failure (Cumming & Cumming, 1957), expressed the dissenting opinion most eloquently:

> What members did not talk about directly was the possibility that the mental health movement is reinforcing a kind of last-ditch individualism which characterizes some aspects of our society. Several times it was mentioned that the movement may just be "pushing middle class norms." Is not the emphasis upon inner harmony and inner happiness an example of an inturned if not a frankly narcissistic, culture? (Quoted in NAMHE, 1960, p. 6)

There was agreement on what mental health is *not*. It is not

1. Adjustment under all our circumstances
2. Freedom from anxiety and tension
3. Freedom from dissatisfaction
4. Conformity
5. Constant harmony
6. A lessening of accomplishment and achievement
7. The absence of personal idiosyncracies
8. The undermining of authority
9. Opposition to religious values

It was also relatively easy for the conferees to develop a classification of mental health educational efforts. Three types were noted: communication to the anonymous individual (via exhibits, posters, leaflets, television, radio, newspapers), communications to a target figure or homogeneous group (patients, retirees, etc.), and communications coupled with action (face-to-face meetings for film or filmstrip showings, plays, or education by group discussion).

An emphasis on early development as a focus for education and on parents as the most likely targets was developed at the 1958 meeting. However, goals for positive mental health were not formulated until the NAMHE contracted with the National Opinion Research Center (NORC) to produce a monograph on positive mental health. The resultant volume by Davis (1965) attempted to go beyond Marie Jahoda's (1958) earlier formulations of positive mental health. Davis's conclusions are worth detailing, since they are directly relevant to current issues in C&E. He writes that nothing emerged from his review that would provide a practical set of actions to recommend to the general population to increase personal adjustment or prevent mental illness. On the other hand, he found the provision of "warmth and affection" in childbearing to be "the single most widely accepted mental health principle in contemporary America" (p. 60). Davis translated this view, which he humourously terms the "thermodynamic theory of emotional development," into four prescriptions:

1. A parent should not "tell a child you don't love him"
2. A parent should show children a great deal of affection
3. A parent should use praise as a technique of control
4. A parent should cultivate his own emotional security, because parental problems make children insecure. (P. 54)

Nonetheless, Davis's diagnosis of impediments to the development of mental health education programs that are empirically grounded is poor. He states:

The major problem is this: *mental health educators have little or nothing specific and practical to tell the public.* In stark generalizations,

1. The so-called principles of mental hygiene are vague slogans rather than strategies of behavior which can be put into practice.
2. The task of research findings is to challenge existing beliefs of laymen ("big cities are bad for mental health") and professionals

("breast-feeding is good for mental health") rather than to add positive generalizations.

3. Environmental and situational stresses play such an important part in determining generalized subjective distress that candid rules for mental health must include such advice as "Do not be poor or ignorant," and "Stay out of armed combat."

4. There is no known method of preventing the major functional psychoses.

5. There are no known rules for influencing the emotional development of children.

6. Although basic research on these matters is increasing in quantity and quality, it is extremely unlikely that the situation will change much in the next decade, since progress will come from gradual accumulations of knowledge, not from a dramatic experimental breakthrough. (Pp. 138-139; emphasis in the original)

Despite convincing evidence to the contrary, Davis ended his review with a note of guarded optimism, recommending continued pursuit of ways to inform the public about adjustment and development. Indeed, he suggests that to do nothing is irresponsible.

Nonetheless, even before Davis's book appeared, informational and educational services were included in P.L. 88-164, a consequence, as Adelson and Lurie (1970) note, of the 1961 *Action for Mental Health* report of the Joint Commission on Mental Illness and Health. There is little evidence to suggest that any of the questions raised by the NAMHE had been adequately resolved, and since the legislative guidelines were so vague (including the 1975 amendments as far as education is concerned), there is no reason to suppose that the controversy about the relative emphasis on mental illness or mental health has ended. Nonetheless, educational programs enjoy current popularity. This may be the result of a current focus of mental health education on demystifying clinical problems and their treatment and on promoting the development of competencies. Another essential factor in understanding the current role of mental health education is the popularity of self-help experiences (books, lectures, workshops) as well as widespread interest in certain psychosocial topics, particularly parenting, psychosocial issues of women, and stress. The interest of the public in knowledge about "normal" life events and life stresses (popularized by Gail Sheehy's *Passages,* for instance) may account for more of the success of CMHC offerings than the programs themselves or their marketing.[7] Certainly, the interest in diverse educational programs is not the result of definitive research on different interventions. In fact, a recent review of self-help behavior therapy manuals (Glasgow & Rosen, 1978) found that the validation of such works is "extremely variable." Thus, the current status of mental health education reflects the same paradox that Davis (1965) provided: despite little objective and empirical evidence for its effectiveness, mental health education remains worth pursuing. Williams (Note 9) makes a convincing case for the cost-effectiveness of mental health education, calling it "the untapped resource." Yet, Bloom's (1980) *Annual Review of Psychology* report questions its mission and purpose, while simultaneously affirming its promise:

> When employed to its fullest, MHE can have significant impact on major segments of the community. In order to realize that potential, however, MHE as a strategy must be understood and implemented. . . . MHE, like all education, is more than the presentation of information. MHE is a process that involves the sharing of information, but much more. (P. 128)

Although there is some question as to whether MHE is indeed a "strategy" as Bloom claims, a definition has recently emerged. As proposed in 1977 by the National Committee for Mental Health Education, mental health education is

> . . .a distinct group of interventions designed to assist people in acquiring knowledge, skills, and attitudes that directly contribute to their mental health and to their effect on the mental health of others. Such interventions enable people to cope with and act on their environment and seek to create environments which are more supportive of human life. MHE is applicable to a wide variety of purposes and target groups, and has unique potential for preventing emotional disability and for promoting growth in people and in community groups. (National Committee for Mental Health Education, Note 10, p. 2)

---

[7]It is interesting to note that the two most popular mental health promoting educative efforts, the Dale Carnegie courses and Gordon's (1970) PET, did not originate in CMHCs nor are they generally acknowledged in the "official" writings on prevention. Price et al.'s (1980) volume on prevention in mental health makes no mention of PET, nor does the Vermont Primary Prevention Conference volume on social competence in children (Kent & Rolf, 1979) nor does Kessler and Albee's pioneering review (1975), except in a passing reference along with such other "interventions" as Zoom, titanium paint, and yogurt!

More specifically, the committee categorized Mental Health Education into five major types:

1. *Education of the General Public*
   — Education about mental health problems and resources
   — Education to promote mental health
2. *Education of "Non-Client, Non-Patient" Populations Which are at Risk*
   — Education to assist people in coping with predictable transitions
   — Education to assist people living under stressful conditions
   — Education to assist people experiencing symptoms of stress
3. *Education of Clients or Patients and Their Significant Others*
   — Education to assist the client in becoming a skilled and knowledgeable consumer of services
   — Education to enhance the therapeutic program of a client or patient
   — Education to facilitate the transition of a client back into the community
4. *Education of Those in the Community who are in a Key Position to Affect the Lives of Others*
5. *Education of Those who are in a Position of Influencing and Effecting Policy.* (National Committee for Mental Health Education, Note 10)

This definition includes *both* mental illness *and* mental health education efforts, recognizing the goals of each as legitimate. The issue of values and morality as stumbling blocks, so volatile an issue in 1956, was not addressed, and major progress in the delineation of positive mental health has not occurred. There have been, on the other hand, considerable advances in the development of mental health educational materials, the two most prominent examples being parenting and social skills training. Much research has yet to be done, however, to demonstrate that even these fairly well designed interventions have a distinct impact on vulnerability reduction (Heller, Price, & Sher, 1980, p. 293).

Mental health education, being an even broader category than consultation, is characterized by national data that are equally sketchy. CMHCs annually report educational activities to NIMH under "Public Information and Public Education," a category defined as follows:

This is a one-way educational process of imparting knowledge to and changing attitudes of the general public, segments of the population, or special target groups to increase understanding of positive mental health and mental disorder and availability of resources. Public information and public education is intended to: 1) increase public awareness of problems found in the community; 2) develop appropriate public action for the alleviation and prevention of such problems; 3) change attitudes, motivations, and behavior; and 4) disseminate information about agencies which provide appropriate human services. It includes such activities as speeches to community organizations, child-rearing classes or workshops for parents, community development activities, etc. Staff hours include preparation as well as activity time. (NIMH, Note 3)

Several problems are inherent with this manner of reporting. First, no distinction is allowed for mental illness prevention versus mental health promotion. Second, approaches that differ widely on many dimensions (a speech versus a parenting program, for example) are treated in the same category. Relatively passive ways of providing information are not separated from complex educational curricula. Third, community development activities, a catch-all that many would assume to be consultative in nature, are out of place. Nonetheless, this is the "E" in NIMH's accounting of C&E activities.

There is little doubt that mental health education efforts will continue, despite the many conceptual and accounting shortcomings. It is also true that the four components of mental health education programs that Davis (1965) noted, namely (1) substantive content, (2) medium or vehicle, (3) audience, and (4) goals, are likely to shift with changing social circumstances and changing interests of both planners and audiences. Regardless of such unpredictable changes in programming, the essential feature of mental health education — its focus on the general public in communities — will remain constant. Exactly which segment of the general public becomes the priority target for education may remain fluid. Erich Lindemann's comment at the 1956 NAMHE meeting is timeless.

We mental health people have a choice of targets for our education. We can concentrate on safeguarding the health of potential victims or we can try to influence administrators and community planners to arrange the situation so as to reduce the number of casualties. The first approach is much more comfortable and satisfying; the second one often gets us into trouble. (Quoted in NAMHE, 1960, p. 63)

A SYNTHESIS OF CURRENT C&E PRACTICE

The histories of mental health consultation and mental health education chronicle sincere efforts by mental health professionals to use technologies that are intrinsically multiplicative in their outcomes. These histories also demonstrate that agreement on *technology* ignores and may even obscure disagreement about *goals*. Toward what end will C&E professionals work? What is the *message* that these powerful techniques transmit to communities? To answer these questions as abstractions ignores the context in which the answers will be played out — the CMHC. The sociopolitical context that supported the development of CMHCs in the 1960s and early 1970s was one in which mental health was broadly defined and the influence of social problems on mental health widely accepted. All signs point to a different context for the CMHCs of the 1980s — one in which fiscal restraint interplays with ideological conservatism. If Levine and Levine's (1970) analysis holds true, it seems likely that the mental health problems will be couched in individualistic versus societal terms. While it is certain that consultation and education will be provided to local catchment areas, the goals of these services will be shaped by state and local funding sources.

Primary prevention has always been a controversial goal for C&E in CMHCs (Perlmutter & Vayda, 1978; Snow & Newton, 1976). It seems likely that it will remain so, despite the arguments for its viability (President's Commission on Mental Health, Task Panel on Prevention, 1978). The relationship of C&E to prevention seems doomed to obfuscation. A recent example can be found in the 1980 NIMH Publication, *Definitions of Terms in Mental Health, Alcohol Abuse, Drug Abuse, and Mental Retardation* (NIMH, Note 6). This publication lists as the universe of services the following: clinical-oriented services, prevention-oriented services, consultation-oriented services, training-oriented services, research-oriented services, and intraorganizational support services. As critiques have pointed out, the definition provided for prevention is in truth a definition of educational services, and the definition of consultation (essentially case consultation) is too limited. More important, the NIMH definition confounds *goals* and *techniques*, a recurrent problem for C&E.

Goals for C&E Services

Because of the repeated confusion of the purposes and goals of C&E and the approaches and techniques used, a framework for C&E services must aid in the clarification of goals. Such a framework must also acknowledge the multiple levels of influence at which C&E energies can be directed. As Rappaport (1977) has noted, the same type of goal can be pursued at differing levels of analysis. C&E programs can have goals that are *promotion* oriented (primary prevention in the typical terminology), *prevention* oriented (early identification or secondary prevention) or can be directed at *rehabilitation* (tertiary prevention or treatment). A useful fourth goal might be *protection* oriented services (defined as "activities or services intended to change laws, regulations, or social structures so that various publics will not be affected by noxious agents or conditions that are believed to be damaging to mental or emotional functioning" (SRB, Note 7, p. 7), such as ordinances prohibiting lead-base paints or law controlling substance abuse. Each of these goals can be seen as legitimate goals for C&E programs, and it is likely that the relative focus of any particular C&E unit can be easily determined.

The *strategies* used to deal with these goals are those typically considered under the C&E rubric. Ketterer and Bader's (Note 2) typology, shown in Table 1-II, provides a list of C&E strategies, essentially a content-free *technology* that can be applied to any goal whether it is protection, promotion, prevention, or rehabilitation (obviously certain strategies are generally more compatible with certain goals).

The final dimension of a C&E framework concerns the *level of analysis* at which the C&E program operates: individual, small group, organizational, and institutional-community (Rappaport, 1977). Any C&E program can be conceived of as an intervention at a specific *level of analysis* pursuing a *goal or intent* using a *technique or strategy*. Figure 1-1 shows hypothetical C&E efforts that emerge when intervention goals are considered at each of the four levels of analysis. These are possible programs that *could* be pursued by C&E units. No prioritizing of goals is assumed; on the contrary, each C&E program must decide how resources will be

Table 1-II
KETTERER AND BADER'S TYPOLOGY OF C&E SERVICES

Services to the Community

1. *Case Consultation:* helping caregivers in other agencies to help their clients achieve treatment goals

2. *Caregiver Consultation and Training:* assisting professionals, paraprofessionals and lay helpers to become more effective in carrying out their respective roles, as well as assisting them in developing ties to relevant professional agencies

3. *Administrative Consultation:* providing technical expertise to community organizations and administrators regarding program design, management, evaluation and organizational development

4. *Program Consultation:* providing technical assistance to community agencies about the content of their programs

5. *Grassroots Consultation:* assisting informal community groups to identify needs, to develop methods for meeting needs, to seek resources and to develop appropriate problem-solving strategies

6. *Network/Coalition Building:* working in interagency or group coalitions to enhance community well-being, to share information and resources and to develop appropriate problem-solving strategies

7. *Public Mental Health Education:* informing the community about services provided by the CMHC and other organizations; changing knowledge/attitudes about mental health through public presentations, literature dissemination, use of media, etc.

8. *Competence Training:* providing in-depth educational training to normal and at-risk groups to increase their problem-solving skills and coping strategies

9. *Community Crisis Intervention:* intervening in community crises to reduce tension and to identify underlying problems/issues

10. *Client Advocacy:* assisting individuals in the community to secure needed resources or support

Services Directed Toward the Mental Health Program

1. *Needs Assessment:* systematically determining community needs for mental health services using a variety of research methods

2. *Information Dissemination to Program:* packaging information for center staff and board, e.g. newsletters, announcements of training programs

3. *Program Staff Development:* planning and providing CMHC in-service training

4. *Evaluation:* monitoring and evaluting centerwide services

5. *Program Board Consultation:* providing information to and assisting CMHC boards in carrying out their functions

6. *Program Staff Meeting Participation:* participating in CMHC meetings, e.g. supervisory sessions, general CMHC staff meetings

7. *Program Planning and Development:* consulting in the development of CMHC policies and procedures; planning and coordinating the delivery of CMHC services

8. *External Committee Work:* representing the CMHC on committees that involve outside agencies (not directly related to C&E activities)

9. *Program Staff Consultation:* consulting with CMHC direct service staff who are delivering consultation/education services

10. *Program Miscellaneous Tasks:* performing other tasks related to the maintenance of the CMHC, e.g. preparing or writing grant proposals that primarily benefit the center

	Levels of Analysis			
	Individual	Small Group	Organizational	Institutional Community
Protection	Client advocacy	Develop program to protect children from family neglect	Promote standards for community living homes for deinstitutionalized	Legal advocacy
Promotion	Assertiveness Training; Goal Setting	Parenting Groups; Training Natural Helpers	Organizational Development; Policy Review	Community Development and Planning
Prevention	Screening Programs	Consultation with Teachers of High-Risk Children	Programs to Divert from Juvenile Justice Systems	Community Coalitions to Reduce Problems
Remediation	MHE on Clinical Services for Adults	Advocacy for Families of Retarded Adults	Troubled Employee Programs in Industry	Community Coalitions to Address Current Problems

Figure 1-1. Goals for Consultation and Education programs.

allocated. C&E is distinguished, in this view, by its commitment to community-based programming and expansion of mental health resources. The technologies that are appropriate to implement these general goals are consultation, training, education, advocacy, use of the media, use of new sources of person power, building of linkages, and so on.

Delivery Systems for C&E Services

All services have an underlying conceptual model and a delivery system (Rappaport & Chinsky, 1974). Because of the diversity of its goals, C&E can and must take advantage of developments that expand the delivery system for mental health services. Fortunately, there have been major advances in this area. The history of mental health over the last two decades reflects a transition from a service system exclusively based on professionals to the current situation in which more than half of direct services are provided by paraprofessionals and nonprofessionals (Task Panel on Personnel, 1978). Even more recently, the notion of who can provide mental health services has extended to local residents without formal attachment to the mental health system, such as members of self-help groups, support groups, and informal community helpers. The trend in mental health has clearly been away from traditional service systems toward helping in least restrictive environments, even to client's homes. Many of these newer forms of help are nonclinical in nature. Therefore, it seems likely to assume that C&E personnel will be involved in liaison, training or supervision of these other helpers (Gershon & Biller, 1977). Since new helpers can, in principle, be used for rehabilitation, prevention, promotion and protection purposes, it may fall to C&E to develop these innovative sources of person-power. The evidence to date suggests that they will be used as treatment adjuncts (e.g. D'Augelli, 1981) unless careful alternative planning is provided (Vallance & D'Augelli, 1982).

Consideration of the diversity of personnel and services results in the typology presented in Figure 1-2. Paraprofessionals are human service workers without advanced degrees; nonprofessionals are workers who are chosen because of their life experiences to function in helping roles within a service system; gatekeepers

	Personnel				
	Paraprofs.	Nonprofs.	Informal Helpers	Gatekeepers	Mass Media
Protection	Use paras to warn of local health problems	Train nonpros to educate women about legal recourse in spouse abuse	Organize local helpers to combat vandalism	Promote lobbying by gatekeepers for protective legislation	Media campaign on children's rights
Promotion	Using paras for mental health education	Decision-making led by nonprofs.	Consulting with support groups of untroubled parents	Train teachers in social competence training	Series on setting life goals and planning
Prevention	Training Head Start personnel to identify hyperactivity	Use of senior citizen counselors to identify high-risk elderly	Groups to inform neighbors of signs of stress and dysfunction	Consult with lawyers to prevent neg. consequences of divorce	Series on critical life events and dealing with consequent stress
Remediation	Mental hospital aide training	Consulting with drug and alcohol counselors	Development of social support for deinstitutionalized persons	Teach police crisis intervention	Series on understanding the "mentally disabled" etc.

Figure 1-2. Consultation and Education service delivery models.

are community persons who serve a mental health function because of close interpersonal contact with others, such as lawyers, police, teachers and religious leaders; informal helpers are the "natural neighbors" who are known as good listeners and problem solvers but have *no* attachment to formal service systems (this includes self-help groups); mass media include print, radio and television. The examples of services given are those that could legitimately fall under the C&E umbrella.

Local planning is necessary to decide how to use these new sources of mental health help. This framework has the essential advantage of separating goals from methods to pursue goals. Since any of the techniques included in Ketterer and Bader's list (Table 1-II) could be used to pursue any of the sixteen goals of Figure 1-1 and tap any combination of the five kinds of service delivery systems, it should come as no surprise that the ostensible tasks of C&E are overwhelming. Many C&E programs are limited in their focus, emphasizing case finding, referral, and public relations for their center. Others are much more ambitious, seeking to implement goals that are promotion or prevention oriented. As example, a CMHC might articulate these goals in the following way:

The Department of C&E develops, implements and maintains programs that promote mental health and prevent mental illness. Specific objectives for this prevention/promotion goal include the following:

1. Enhancing prenatal development
2. Enhancing parents' ability to raise their children
3. Enhancing individual's ability to cope with normal life challenges
4. Better preparing individuals for natural high stress periods
5. Developing improved support for persons currently experiencing high stress
6. Enhancing the professional and lay community of helpers
7. Developing community systems and policies that facilitate growth
8. Developing community attitudes that support positive mental health.

Regardless of the breadth or narrowness of programming in any particular C&E program, it seems useful to consider the relative emphasis on different mental health goals and the value positions that are implicit.

Problems

Despite the clear mandate for C&E services, the incredible variety of programming that can be provided by C&E personnel, and the increased sophistication of those in the C&E area, C&E has yet to achieve prominence as a mental health service (Yolles, 1977). Ketterer and Bader's (Note 2) analysis details five major areas that can account for this situation:

1. C&E has never received the resources necessary to complete its mandate.
2. There has been a lack of adequate federal guidelines for C&E including a lack of a typology of services, a failure to clarify the relationship of C&E to prevention and promotion, a failure to define criteria of setting program priorities, and a failure to specify minimum CMHC resources for C&E.
3. There has not been a careful effort to develop knowledge about critical dimensions of C&E services.
4. There is little training available for C&E.
5. There has not been adequate documentation and evaluation of C&E services.

Thus, there are major issues to be resolved in fiscal support, conceptual frameworks, the development of a relevant knowledge base, professional education and training and evaluation. These will be briefly discussed.

Fiscal Issues

It is difficult to determine how much federal money has actually been spent on C&E activities. Using NIMH figures, Swift (1980) estimates that 4.1 percent of the federal staffing grant monies for 1965-1978 ($6,300,600 of a total of $1,236,600,006) was for C&E staffing. During this period, however, the number of CMHCs more than doubled (there were 286 in 1967 and 563 in 1978). Also, the 4.1 multiplier is a rather crude figure itself, based on the staff hours spent for C&E over a five-year period (1973-1977) that does not correspond to the expenditure period. Not only is the figure rough, but it also obscures the decreasing trend of C&E staff funding from 1973 to 1977. Other federal funding data reviewed by Swift may be more interpretable, such as the amount of $28,500,000 that was spent between 1976-1979 for special C&E grants. However, this too is imprecise because it covers a four-year period, and not all CMHCs receive these grants. Perhaps the most simple index of support for C&E lies in the allocation of staff hours. On this variable, there has been a gradual but distinctive decline from few to very few hours for C&E. This decline may be partially a function of the expiration of staffing grants, which Swift (1980) notes generally result in C&E services being the first cut. In a similar way, it is possible that this drop can also reflect a reassignment of some C&E staff to clinical services.

The most pressing fiscal problem for C&E has been its non-revenue-generating nature. In 1977, C&E services generated .4 percent of the funds for the 563 CMHCs (NIMH, Note 8), whereas direct services generated 35.7 percent of the revenue. The need for C&E to pursue outside reimbursement can lead to several outcomes: (1) only C&E services that generate fees would be provided, with resources such as middle class parents or wealthier school districts; (2) fewer C&E services that are promotion oriented would be offered. Educational programs will be recast as therapeutic events so as to qualify for insurance payment; (3) only individuals who can do clinical work and C&E would be hired for staff positions, essentially forcing mental health educators, policy analysts, and program specialists to "cover their bets" with clinical training; (4) little effort would be directed to pressing problematic social conditions, since challenges to the status quo do not generate anything except controversy; and (5) collaboration with nonclinical helpers in the community (self-help groups, support groups, natural helpers) would be curtailed if not eliminated. It is certainly true that C&E staff can be more creative and aggressive in pursuing local sources of support for programs, and it is possible to seek out private sources of funds such as philanthropies and business. Yet, it remains unclear whether or not C&E units can survive a "fee for service" ideology in which programs exist only if they are self-supporting. Federal legislation, perhaps more than any other variable, will have a major influence. The Mental Health Systems Act[8] includes a provision for grants to support "nonrevenue producing activities," a clear recognition that some community mental health services will not generate a positive cash flow. Without such recognition, consultation, education and prevention are likely to be curtailed drastically. While such a course would not necessarily lead to the demise of C&E, it would result in a reorientation toward clinically oriented C&E services at the sacrifice of prevention.

Conceptual Issues

On a conceptual level, consultation, education and prevention suffers from diffuse boundaries, and no agreed-upon domain yet exists. Many of the typologies described in this chapter delimit C&E, and there are general conceptual frameworks that can also direct C&E planning. For prevention planning, Dohrenwend (1978) describes a model linking psychological and situational events with stressful life events and their consequences. Albee (1980) provides an equation for problematic behavior in which stress and constitutional vulnerabilities are balanced by the psychosocial resources of social support, coping skills and competence. A similar, more complex, model of psychosocial stress is provided by Snow and Blackford (Note 12), and Snow and Swift (Note 13) cite implications of the model for primary prevention.

For promotion planning, a colleague and I (Danish & D'Augelli, 1980) have recently described a *human development intervention* model of services that avoids some of the pitfalls that are inherent in remediation and prevention. This model stresses the need for an understanding of normative individuals and family development, an analysis of expected and unexpected life events as points of intervention, and the development of an array of services that are as ecologically relevant as possible. (This is the human development equivalent of least restrictive environment.)

---

[8] As of this writing, the status of the Mental Health Systems Act in unclear. Passed by Congress in 1980, its implementation was delayed. The concept of "block grants" to states for mental health and other services, and a trend toward local control, question what role NIMH will play in the future of CMHCs. The fate of C&E services should the Systems Act be repealed is even more uncertain. Since most initiatives for prevention have been at the national level, it seems unlikely that C&E will receive even the modest financial support it has to date.

Since a human development approach embodies all the levels of analysis that Rappaport (1977) has described, programming can accomplish broader goals of creating a competent community (Iscoe, 1974). A recent project designed to increase the helpfulness in communities by enhancing helping networks (D'Augelli, Vallance, Danish, Young & Gerdes, 1981) provides one example of the model in use. The promotion perspective of a human development model can be found elsewhere as well, for example, in relationship enhancement (Guerney, 1977), social competence training (Spivack & Shure, 1974), self-help groups (Gartner & Reissman, 1977), support groups for life crises, and so on. C&E programs can incorporate two prime goals with this model: the modification of social environments and the promotion of life skills (Cowen, 1973).

Knowledge Base Issues

To a great degree, the issue of knowledge about C&E services depends on the nature of C&E in the future. Some prototypical C&E services have, contrary to Ketterer and Bader's conclusion, been subject to extensive research. Examples are Cowen's model for early identification and treatment of school problems (Cowen, Trost, Izzo, Lorion, Dorr & Issacson, 1975), Spivack and Shure's social problem solving (Spivack & Shure, 1974; Urbain & Kendall, 1980), training in relationship-enhancing skills (Guerney, 1977), and training in helping skills (Danish, D'Augelli & Brock, 1976). Much empirical work is accumulating on informal helping and social support (see Heller, 1979, and Mitchell & Trickett, 1980, for reviews) and on the stresses of everyday life (Dohrenwend & Dohrenwend, 1974). Conversely, our knowledge of C&E per se is remarkably meager. Ketterer and Bader's (Note 2) study is an excellent example of the kind of investigation needed on a national level. We may have some encouraging evidence about what kinds of programs "work" (at least, in a limited sense) but we know little about what is currently being provided by C&E. Unfortunately, as this analysis has shown, the NIMH data are not useful for this purpose.

Training Issues

Professional issues blocking C&E are considerable. Specific training is not available for C&E, and continuing education is minimal, despite the valiant efforts of the Staff College of NIMH and regional and state organizations. National or regional organizations representing C&E are beginning to emerge, and a national C&E conference now exists. However, poor preparation and training, inadequate support at the local level, and the consequent turnover of personnel have continued to take the allure from C&E positions. This may change if and when C&E gains an identity as a distinct set of orientations and services for which specific training is essential. A further need may be differentiated C&E functions for different levels of training personnel. While a master's degree is the modal degree for C&E staff, the demands of program development and evaluation are such that doctoral training may be suggested for C&E directors. C&E's lack of a clear attachment to a specific mental health professional discipline may be a weakness, but it is also a source of strength, reflecting the unique interdisciplinary nature of C&E services.

Evaluation Issues

The documentation of C&E programs has been a persistent problem, as the analysis of NIMH's attempts at accounting show. When some agreed-upon set of definitions emerges (SRED's [Note 7] is the most fruitful set to date), it is possible that the simple act of description can proceed. This must occur before hard evaluative questions can be posed. However, program evaluation is impeded if goals are unclear. In a detailed critique of the evaluation of consultation programs, Jerrel and Schulberg (1981) write:

> Obstacles to rigorous specification of C&E goals include the lack of a clear administrative mandate, the failure of consultants to assess baseline target behaviors or misperceptions, and inability of C&E directors to translate information regarding "need" into a service with operationalized objectives and activities. . . . A majority of program managers do not conduct a systematic needs assessment. They, therefore, are unable to specify clear-cut program goals, well-delineated clients and anticipated outcomes which can be assessed through appropriate evaluation procedures. (P. 7)

CONCLUSIONS

C&E services are in transition. Long a part of CMHCs, C&E has the intense national interest in prevention in mental health as its current ally. As Albee (1980) suggests, prevention may indeed be the fourth mental health revolution. However, the revolution finds its natural proponents, C&E personnel, in a state of disarray and disorder. C&E professionals must address the current image of C&E as adjunctive to clinical services; must delineate C&E's distinct identity, goals, resources and needs; and must work to develop innovative ways of involving the community in C&E activities. C&E must not lose the opportunity to direct the revolution. On the other hand, C&E must insure that the benefits of the revolution do not accrue only to the middle class, a potential consequence of the fiscal pressures that CMHCs and their C&E units face.

The mandate for C&E is nothing if not overwhelming. No other mental health service is trying to accomplish so much with so little. No other mental health service is without a tradition of its own to call on or lacks a history of common practices and professional wisdom. No other service modality seems as subject to the forces of government funding and guidelines. Caught between the treatment-oriented structure of the CMHC and an ideological commitment to *community* mental health, C&E is vulnerable to the winds of change. This vulnerability may be fatal if shifting federal priorities exclude C&E services. Being more positive, this vulnerability may be a critical stimulus for C&E professionals to clarify their goals. For example, the interest in primary prevention and promotion may well be ephemeral, extinguished by half-hearted efforts that have little visibility or impact. Prevention may be the mental health equivalent of the War on Poverty, a program of lofty liberal goals that was haphazardly implemented and poorly evaluated, thus leading to a historical judgment that the effort was intrinsically flawed. It would indeed be tragic if social critics in the 1990s look back on C&E as a misguided effort to reach an impossible goal. A coherent attempt to resolve issues facing C&E is required to maintain the eroding momentum of the commitment to community mental health during the 1980s.

In a basic sense, optimism about the future of C&E is justified. Mental health is a volatile, yet lasting commodity in the human service marketplace. At the National Assembly on Mental Health Education, one of the conferees, the Reverend C. Leslie Glenn, provided this witty insight into the breadth of mental health issues in our culture:

> Half the world is engaged in helping the other half find mental health. Even bank advertisements don't promise to guard your money, but to give you peace of mind. (Quoted in NAMHE, p. ix)

ANNOTATED REFERENCES

1. Howery, V. I. Working paper on Consultation and Education — Definitions and Concepts. Prepared by Task Force on C&E, National Council of Community Mental Health Centers, February, 1976.

2. Ketterer, R. F., & Bader, B. C. Issues in the development of consultation and education services in community mental health centers. Michigan Department of Mental Health Report, December, 1977. Available from Center for Human Services Research, P.O. Box 2167, Ann Arbor, MI 48106.

3. National Institute of Mental Health. Provisional data on federally funded community mental health centers (annual report). Available from Survey and Reports Branch, Division of Biometry and Epidemiology, NIMH, 5600 Fishers Lane, Room 18C17, Rockville, MD 20852.

4. Hassler, F. Overview of the national C&E data. Unpublished report available from Ferdinand Hassler, Staff College — NIMH, 5635 Fishers Lane, Rockville, MD 20852.

5. Klein, D. C. Criteria for selecting C&E staff and staff development for C&E programming. Paper prepared for NIMH Staff College, n.d. Available from F. Hassler (see Note 4).

6. National Institute of Mental Health. Definitions for use in mental health information systems. DHEW Publication No. (ADM) 80-833, 1980.

7. Southern Regional Education Board. Definitions for prevention/promotion services in mental health. Unpublished report, 1980. Available from SREB, 130 Sixth Street, N.W., Atlanta, GA 30313.

8. National Institute of Mental Health. Provisional data on federally funded community mental health centers, 1977-1978. See note 3.

9. Williams, R. T. Mental health education: The untapped resource. Paper developed for the Michigan Mental Health Association. Available from R. T. Williams, University of Wisconsin-Extension, 610 Langdon Street, Madison, WI 53706.

10. National Committee for Mental Health Education. Mental health education: A concept paper. March, 1977.

11. Bass, R. D., & Rosenstein, M. The indirect services: Consultation and education and public information and public education, federally funded community mental health centers. Mental Health Statistical Note No. 147. Survey and Reports Branch, Division of Biometry and Epidemiology. See Note 3 for address.

12. Snow, D. L., & Blackford, V. A psychosocial model of stress. Unpublished manuscript, 1978. Available from D. L. Snow, Yale University of Medicine, 24 Part Street, New Haven, CT 06519.

13. Snow, D.L., & Swift, C. Consultation and education: Definition and Philosophy. Unpublished manuscript, n.d.

BIBLIOGRAPHY

1. Adelson, D., & Lurie, L. Mental health education: Research and practice. In S. E. Golann & C. Eisdorfer (Eds.), *Handbook of community mental health.* New York: Appleton-Century-Crofts, 1972.

2. Albee, G. W. Prevention in community mental health centers. In H. S. Resnick, C. Ashton, & C. S. Palley (Eds.), *The health care system and drug abuse prevention.* Washington, D.C.: NIDA, 1980.

3. Baizerman, M., & Hall, W. T. Consultation as a political process. *Community Mental Health Journal,* 1977, *13,* 142-149.

4. Berlin, I. N. Some learning experiences as a psychiatric consultant to schools. *Mental Hygiene,* 1956, *40,* 215-236.

5. ———. Learning mental health consultation — history and problems. *Mental Hygiene,* 1964, *48,* 257-267.

6. ———. Some lessons learned in 25 years of mental health consultation to schools. In S. C. Plog & P. I Ahmed (Eds.), *Principles and techniques of mental health consultation.* New York: Plenum, 1977.

7. Bloom, B. L. Social and community interventions. *Annual Review of Psychology,* 1980, *31,* 111-142.

8. Caplan, G. *Principles of preventive psychiatry.* New York: Basic Books, 1964.

    ———. *The theory and practice of mental health consultation.* New York: Basic Books, 1970.

9. ———. Mental health consultation: Retrospect and prospect. In S. C. Plog & P. I. Ahmed (Eds.), *Principles and techniques of mental health consultation.* New York: Plenum, 1977.

10. Caplan, R. B. *Helping the helpers to help.* New York: Seabury Press, 1972.

11. Cherness, C. Preentry issues in consultation. *American Journal of Community Psychology,* 1976, *4,* 13-24.

12. ———. Creating new consultation programs in community mental health centers: Analysis of a case study. *Community Mental Health Journal,* 1977, *13,* 133-141.

13. Collins, A. H., & Pancoast, D. L. *Natural helping networks.* Washington: NASW, 1976.
14. Cowen, E. L. Social and community interventions. *Annual Review of Psychology,* 1973, *24,* 423-472.
15. Cowen, E. L., Trost, M. A., Izzo, L. D., Lorion, R. P., Dorr, D., & Isaacson, R. V. *New ways in school mental health.* New York: Human Sciences, 1975.
16. Cumming, E., & Cumming, J. *Closed ranks: An experiment in mental health education.* Cambridge: Harvard University Press, 1957.
17. Danish, S. J., & D'Augelli, A. R. Promoting competence and enhancing development through life development intervention. In L. A. Bond & J. C. Rosen (Eds.), *Primary prevention of psychopathology* (Vol. 4). Hanover, N.H.: University Press of New England, 1980.
18. Danish, S. J., D'Augelli, A. R., & Brock, G. W. An evaluation of helping skills training: Effects on helpers' verbal responses. *Journal of Counseling Psychology,* 1976, *23,* 259-266.
19. D'Augelli, A. R. Future directions for paraprofessionals in rural mental health, or how to avoid giving indigenous helpers civil service ratings. In P. A. Keller & J. D. Murray (Eds.), *Handbook of rural community mental health.* New York: Human Sciences Press, 1981.
20. D'Augelli, A. R., Vallance, T. R., Danish, S. J., Young, C. E., & Gerdes, J. R. The Community Helpers Project: A description of a prevention strategy for rural communities. *Journal of Prevention,* 1981.
21. Davis, J. A. *Education for positive mental health.* Chicago: Aldine, 1965.
22. Dohrenwend, B. S. Social stress and community psychology. *American Journal of Community Psychology,* 1978, *6,* 1-14.
23. Dohrenwend, B. S., & Dohrenwend, B. (Eds.), *Stressful life events.* New York: Wiley, 1974.
24. Dworkin, A. L., & Dworkin, E. P. A conceptual overview of selected consultation models. *American Journal of Community Psychology,* 1975, *3,* 151-159.
25. Gartner, A., & Reissman, F. *Self-help in the human services.* San Francisco: Jossey-Bass, 1978.
26. Glasgow, R. E., & Rosen, G. M. Behavioral bibliotherapy: A review of self-help behavior therapy manuals. *Psychological Bulletin,* 1978, *85,* 1-23.
27. Gershon, M., & Biller, H. B. *The other helpers.* Lexington, Mass.: Lexington, 1977.

28. Grady, M. A., Gibson, M. S., & Trickett, E. J. *Mental health consultation theory, practice, and research, 1973-1978.* (DHHS Publication No. (ADM) 81-948). Washington, D. C.: U. S. Government Printing Office, 1981.

29. Guerney, B. G. *Relationship enhancement.* San Francisco: Jossey-Bass, 1977.

30. Hassol, L., & Cooper, S. Mental health consultation in a preventive context. In H. Grunebaum (Ed.), *The practice of community mental health.* Boston: Little Brown, 1970.

31. Heck, E. T., Gomez, A. G., & Adams, G. L. *A guide to mental health services.* Pittsburgh: University of Pittsburgh Press, 1973.

32. Heller, K. The effects of social support: Prevention and treatment implications. In A. P. Goldstein & F. H. Kanfer (Eds.), *Maximizing treatment gains.* New York: Academic Press, 1979.

33. Heller, K., & Monahan, J. *Psychology and community change.* Homewood, Ill.: Dorsey, 1977.

34. Heller, K., Price, R. H., & Sher, K. J. Research and evaluation in primary prevention. In R. H. Price, R. F. Ketterer, C. B. Bader, & Monahan, J. (Eds.), *Prevention in mental health.* Beverly Hills, CA: Sage, 1980.

35. Iscoe, I. Community psychology and the competent community. *American Psychologist,* 1974, *29,* 607-613.

36. Jahoda, M. *Current concepts of positive mental health.* New York: Basic Books, 1958.

37. Jerrell, J. M., & Schulberg, H. C. The evaluation of mental health consultation programs. In H. Goldstein & S. Feldman (Eds.), *Mental health consultation: Principles and practices.* New York: Neale Watson Academic Publications, 1981.

38. Kelly, J. G. The quest for valid preventive interventions. In C. D. Spielberger (Ed.), *Current topics in community and clinical psychology* (Vol. 2). New York: Academic Press, 1970.

39. Kent, M. W., & Rolf, J. E. (Eds.), *Primary prevention of psychopathology: Social competence in children.* (Vol. III) Hanover, N.H.: University Press of New England, 1979.

40. Kessler, M., & Albee, G. W. Primary prevention. *Annual Review of Psychology,* 1975, *26,* 557-591.

41. Lepkin, M. A program of industrial consultation by a community mental health center. *Community Mental Health Journal,* 1975, *11,* 74-81.

42. Levine, M., & Levine, A. *Social history of the helping services.* New York: Appleton-Century-Crofts, 1970.

43. Lindemann, E. Symptomatology and management of acute grief. *American Journal of Psychiatry,* 1944, *101,* 141-148.

44. Maclennan, B. W. Mental health consultation programs: Priority setting and funding. In A. S. Rogawski (Ed.), *Mental health consultation in community settings*. San Francisco: Jossey Bass, 1979.

45. Mannino, F. V., Maclennan, B. W., & Shore, M. F. *The practice of mental health consultation*. New York: Gardner Press, 1975.

46. Mannino, F. V., & Shore, M. F. Evaluation of consultation: Problems and prospects. In A. S. Rogawski (Ed.), *Mental health consultation in community settings*. San Francisco: Jossey-Bass, 1979.

47. Mazade, N. A. Consultation and education practice and organizational structure in ten community mental health centers. *Hospital and Community Psychology*, 1974, *25*, 673-675.

48. Meyers, J., Parsons, R. D., & Martin, R. *Mental health consultation in the schools*. San Francisco: Jossey-Bass, 1979.

49. Miller, F. T., Mazade, N. A., Muller, S., & Andrulis, D. Trends in community mental health programming. *American Journal of Community Psychology*, 1978, *6*, 191-198.

50. Mitchell, R. E., & Trickett, E. J. Social network research and psychosocial adaptation: Implications for community mental health practice. In P. Insel (Ed.), *Climate of mental health: Perspectives in prevention*. Lexington, Mass.: D. C. Heath, 1980.

51. National Assembly on Mental Health Education. *Mental health education: A critique*. Philadelphia: Author, 1960.

52. Perlmutter, F. Prevention and treatment: A strategy for survival. *Community Mental Health Journal*, 1974, *10*, 276-281.

53. Perlmutter, F., & Silverman, H. A. Conflict in consultation-education. *Community Mental Health Journal*, 1973, *9*, 116-122.

54. Perlmutter, F. D., & Vayda, A. M. Barriers to prevention programs in community mental health centers. *Administration in Mental Health*, 1978, *5*, 140-153.

55. Plog, S. C., & Ahmed, P. I. The common basis of consultation. In S. C. Plog & P. I. Ahmed (Eds.), *Principles and techniques of mental health consultation*. New York: Plenum, 1977.

56. Price, R. H., Ketterer, R. F., Bader, B. C., & Monahan, J. (Eds.), *Prevention in mental health*. Beverly Hills, CA: Sage, 1980.

57. Rappaport, J. *Community psychology*. New York: Holt, 1977.

58. Rappaport, J., & Chinskey, J. M. Models for delivery of service from a historical and conceptual perspective. *Professional Psychology*, 1974, *5*, 42-50.

59. Reinking, R. H., Livesay, G., & Kohl, M. The effects of consultation style on consultee productivity. *American Journal of Community Psychology*, 1978, *6*, 283-290.

60. Reppucci, N. D., Sarata, B. P. V., Saunders, J. T., McArthur, A. V., & Michlin, L. We bombed in Mountville: Lessons learned in consultation to a correctional facility for adolescent offenders. In I. I. Goldenberg (Ed.), *The helping professions in the world of action.* Lexington, Mass.: Lexington, 1973.

61. Signall, K. A., & Scott, P. A. Mental health consultation: An interaction model. *Community Mental Health Journal,* 1971, *7,* 288-302.

62. Snow, D. L., & Newton, P. M. Task, social structure, and social process in the community mental health movement. *American Psychologist,* 1976, *31,* 582-594.

63. Spivack, E., & Shure, M. B. *The social adjustment of young children.* San Francisco: Jossey-Bass, 1974.

64. Swift, C. F. Primary prevention: Policy and practice. In R. H. Price, R. F. Ketterer, C. B. Bader, & Monahan, J. (Eds.), *Prevention in mental health.* Beverly Hills, CA: Sage, 1980.

65. Task Panel on Personnel, *President's Commission on Mental Health.* Washington, D. C.: U.S. Government Printing Office, 1978.

66. Task Panel on Prevention, *President's Commission on Mental Health.* Washington, D.C.: U.S. Government Printing Office, 1978.

67. Urbain, E. S., & Kendall, P. C. Review of social-cognitive problem-solving interventions with children. *Psychological Bulletin,* 1980, *88,* 109-143.

68. Vallance, T. R., & D'Augelli, A. R. The professional as developer of natural helping systems: Conceptual, organizational, and pragmatic considerations. In D. Biegel & A. Naparstek (Eds.), *Community support systems and mental health: Building linkages.* New York: Springer, 1982.

69. Yolles, S. F. A critical appraisal of community mental health services. In G. Serban (Ed.), *New trends of psychiatry in the community.* Cambridge: Ballinger, 1977.

Appendix A

RECIPIENTS OF MENTAL HEALTH CONSULTATION

1. State and local law enforcement and correctional agencies:
   a. representatives of the court, i.e. judges, lawyers, parole agents
   b. police, sheriff's office, highway patrol, etc.
   c. administration and/or staff of penal institutions of training schools
   d. corrections personnel and groups engaged in the rehabilitation of convicts
   e. personnel from professional and citizen groups engaged in planning, research or education with respect to crime delinquency or law enforcement
2. Programs and organizations concerned with alcoholism, includes clubs, organizations, etc.:
   a. servicing alcoholics, e.g. Alcoholics Anonymous, Alateen, etc.
   b. engaged in planning, research or education with respect to the problems of alcoholism
   c. includes employers concerned with alcoholic employees
3. Programs and organizations concerned with other drug abuse:
   a. serving drug abusers (methadone clinics, halfway or residential treatment programs, etc.)
   b. engaged in planning, research or education with respect to the problems of drug abuse
   c. includes employers concerned with employees with drug problems
4. Programs and organizations concerned with family planning: Planned Parenthood, abortion clinics, genetic counseling clinics and programs dealing with human sexuality and sex education.
5. Mental health organizations not affiliated with the organization:
   a. organizations providing direct clinical-oriented services, e.g. state hospitals, family service programs, hot lines, etc.
   b. organizations engaged in planning, research, education or the coordination of service delivery, e.g. NIMH, state boards, and coordinating agencies

6. Health services delivery system:
   a. those providing medical care and physical rehabilitation, e.g. general hospitals, American Red Cross, Public Health Nursing, etc.
   b. those engaged in planning, research, administration, education or coordination of medical services, e.g. Comprehensive Health Planning Agencies, American Hospital Association, etc.
7. Public welfare organizations: Include all that administer, plan and/or provide welfare, e.g. Food Stamp Programs, County Welfare Departments, etc.
8. Programs and organizations for the aged:
   a. those serving the aged, e.g., nursing homes, senior citizen residences, etc.
   b. those engaged in planning, research or education with respect to the elderly
9. Programs and organizations concerned with children (other than schools):
   a. those serving children, e.g. residential facilities, adoption agencies, runaway houses, etc.
   b. those engaged in planning or research with respect to children
10. General public and organizations not classified above include: clubs such as the Jaycees, Kiwanis, Lions Club and church groups.
11. Public and private primary and secondary schools, colleges and universities.
12. Churches and church-related organizations.
13. Business and industry and employment-related organizations (Vocational Rehabilitation, Department of Labor).
14. Governmental policymakers, e.g. legislators, governmental administrators, county commissioners, members of city councils.
15. Self-help and mutual support groups.
16. Community and neighborhood agencies, (e.g. neighborhood planning groups, community action programs, neighborhood associations.

Source: 1-11 from NIMH (Note 6); 12-16 from SREB (Note 7).

Appendix B

TYPES OF MENTAL HEALTH CONSULTATION

A. *Problem-Oriented Consultation:* a process of interaction between a consultant (member of the organization) and a consultee (individual practitioner, agency or institution) outside of the provider organization designed to impart knowledge, increase skill levels and insight and/or modify attitudes such that the consultee is better able to resolve his problems and carry out service responsibilities.

Within the problem-oriented consultation dimension are three major categories. These include case, staff and program consultation. The distinguishing factor among the subcategories is their orientation; that is, all consultations typically have some degree of care, staff or program-related content. However, it is the primary intention, focus or "orientation" of the consultation service delivery that delineates the category.

1. *Case consultation:* services that are designed to assist a consultee in the provision of services (assessment, treatment, and disposition) for a specific client (individual, couple or family) of the consultee. Case-oriented consultation is not considered to be a direct clinical service and purposely excludes instances where the consultant collaborates with the consultee in the direct provision of services to a client. In other words, when the consultant's role extends beyond an advisory relationship to assist the consultee, as is often the case in medical or psychological consultations, the service should be considered and recorded as a direct clinical service.

2. *Staff consultation:* services that are designed to assist a consultee to increase knowledge, improve skill level and/or modify the attitude of the consultee himself. These services are delivered to remedy a lack of skill in the consultee himself or assist in the resolution of an emotional crisis precipitated by the interaction between the consultee's client and himself. This category is intended for use with consultation to a consultee and not treatment. In instances where a professional is in need of treatment services, if services are rendered they

should be recorded as direct clinical work. This category also excludes work with students on internships or practicum placements and in-service training work for the organization itself.

3. *Program consultation:* services that are designed to assist the consultee in the innovation, planning, developing, and implementing of his programs or in solving problems and addressing concerns in his own organization. The main focus is the consultee's programs, services, and activities. These efforts may relate to concern with program administration including planning, policy determination, training, operating efficiency, use of personnel, etc. or concern with intra-agency relations that may have an adverse effect on the provision of services.

B. *Planning and Development-oriented Consultation:* assistance to community organizations, planning organizations, and citizen groups, in planning for the enhancement and enrichment of the community and to develop solutions for community problems through the provision of comprehensive health care services. Planning and development-oriented consultation involves the direct participation of the consultant with others in the planning, developing and innovation process. The consultant representing his organization may be one of many community organizations or agencies involved. It should be noted that these services exclude participation as a private citizen and are limited to those in which the consultant is officially representing his organization. It should be further noted that this category differs from program-oriented consultation in the sense that it focused on *inter*organizational relationships and development, while program-oriented consultation focuses on issues restricted to specific *intra*organizational problems and development.

Source: NIMH (Note 6)

Chapter 2

ORGANIZATIONAL DEVELOPMENT OF CONSULTATION AND EDUCATION

DAVID R. RITTER

THE development of viable Consultation and Education programs within community mental health centers requires examination of both the *structure* and *function* of the program. While considerable attention is often paid to functional aspects, meaning services that will actually be delivered through consultation or education approaches, the organizational structure of C&E is all too often overlooked. This chapter will focus on structural program characteristics necessary for the development of the Consultation and Education program including alternative organizational models, their strengths and weaknesses, and a number of critical issues that can either enhance or impede effective program development.

THE STRUCTURAL FOUNDATION

The organizational structure of the Consultation and Education program, and the foundation upon which it rests, will determine the program's vitality and stability. The building of the C&E program should be analogous to the building of a house. The initial phase of construction is the pouring of the foundation and, only after this has been firmly established, does the phase of the staging of the structure itself begin. If the foundation is weak, the structure is jeopardized, no matter how well designed or thoughtfully planned. When both foundation and structure are sound, the building will have longevity, retaining its stability over time even though its occupants may change.

The foundation for the Consultation and Education program rests not with its philosophical orientation, as philosophy is really linked to services, but rather in the support it has received from the center director and governing board. Support must be strong from these individuals in order for the foundation of the C&E program to have strength. Both the governing board and the center director must demonstrate their commitment to C&E in both word and action. These individuals must believe in the intrinsic value of consultation and education activities as a means of promoting the mental health of the community and must be willing to allocate the necessary resources to sustain this belief. When such a commitment on the part of the center director and the governing board exists, then Consultation and Education has the potential to become a meaningful and integral component of the mental health center. ·If, however, a strong level of commitment is not forthcoming, then the C&E program will likely become a low priority program that exists almost solely to satisfy federal mandates. When one considers that only about 5 percent of all CMHC staff time nationally is devoted to C&E activities, it becomes apparent that compliance with federal guidelines is frequently the main impetus behind the development of Consultation and Education.

How can one determine whether a viable foundation exists for the development of Consultation and Education? An initial determination can be made through an assessment of the inherent beliefs and the verbal statements of the center director and governing board.

Who actually proposed the development of C&E? If the proposal was initially made by the center director or the governing board, then support could be considered to be greater than if the proposal came from one or more staff members of the center.

Why was such a proposal made? It is at this point that one must attempt to ascertain whether the proposal is simply to meet federal mandates that C&E services exist or whether the proposal is offered in response to an identified community need.

What is the current understanding of C&E on the part of the center director and governing board? Indeed, the term Consultation and Education is perhaps one of the most ill-defined concepts within community mental health today.[1] Admittedly, this definition problem may be a difficult one to address. Yet, it should be apparent whether the proposed C&E service would focus on prevention, early intervention or outreach clinical services. Some of the question of *what* may be clarified through a discussion of the target populations within the community that would become the focus for C&E services and why there is a perceived need for services on the part of those target populations.

How might a developed C&E program integrate or conflict with the existing programs of the agency? How much experience, if any, does the center director or staff have in the area of C&E? On a preliminary basis, how much stature would the C&E program have in relationship to other clinical programs of the center?

When should the C&E program begin to be developed? This question is no less important than any of the other questions that have been explored, and it is at this point that reality frequently intrudes upon the ideal. Programs are not developed and implemented overnight. There is much groundwork that needs to be established and planning that needs to occur. The question of *when* will, once again, clarify some of the purposes and expectations surrounding the development of Consultation and Education. It is at this time that an assessment can be made of the depth of the commitment to C&E on the part of the center director and the governing board. Support for a thought-out and well-planned development of C&E represents a greater level of commitment than would be the case of expectations for an immediate program. If there is a push to develop C&E quickly, perhaps to exploit a political opportunity or respond to a very vocal

---

[1] At the 1981 Meeting of The National Council of Community Mental Health Centers, a detailed set of Guidelines for Consultation and Education was proposed by the Council on Prevention and approved by the NCCMHC. These *Recommended Policies and Procedures for Consultation and Education Services Within Community Mental Health Systems/Agencies* can be obtained from the NCCMHC, 2233 Wisconsin Avenue, N.W., Washington, D.C. 20007.

segment of the community to bolster the community mental health center's public image, then insufficient commitment may well exist.

The importance of the development of a firm foundation for Consultation and Education cannot be overemphasized. This foundation cannot rest with one individual, even if it is the center director, as individuals come and go. Instead, the foundation must have breadth, and over time, the commitment to C&E must become part of the community mental health center's purpose for being. On a pragmatic level, the issue of financial resources for the C&E program cannot be overlooked. Allocation of monies tends to coincide with levels of commitment. When commitment exists, monies will follow to support it. Therefore, it is also during this important foundation stage that the financial stability and support of the Consultation and Education program is initially explored.

THE ORGANIZATIONAL STRUCTURE

Once the foundation for the Consultation and Education program has been well established, it is time to consider the organizational structure itself. Essentially, there are three structural models:

— The Centralized C&E Model, which is a distinct organizational unit within the community mental health center with its own director and staff whose sole responsibility is the delivery of consultation and education services.

— The Decentralized C&E Model in which C&E is a quasi-organizational entity having its own coordinator but staffed by individuals whose primary function and identity is with other clinical programs, but who also devote a percentage of time to C&E activities.

— The Mixed C&E Model, which combines aspects of both the Centralized and the Decentralized concepts, having its own director or coordinator, some full-time C&E staff, and some staff time of individuals from other programs of the center.

A review of recent literature on the organizational structures and staffing patterns of Consultation and Education programs within community mental health centers has identified a number of variables that relate closely with the type of organizational structure adopted for the Consultation and Education program. Perlmutter (1979) in a review of Consultation and Education programs within Region III (Delaware, Pennsylvania, Maryland, Virginia, Washington, D.C. and West Virginia) found that centers within rural catchment areas tended to adopt a Decentralized C&E Model, while centers within nonrural catchment areas tended to employ Centralized C&E units. Nine out of every ten of the nonrural centers surveyed did have an organizational unit for Consultation and Education, predominately a Centralized Model approach. This is in contrast to the finding that better than half of the rural community mental health centers surveyed did not have any formalized C&E program. Instead, many rural centers employed an ad hoc approach in which responsibility for C&E services was neither assigned nor allocated to any particular staff but that some staff did, nevertheless, venture into C&E activities.

A preconference survey conducted as part of the First Annual Region I Consultation and Education Conference (Rabow and Rabow, 1978) supported many of Perlmutter's findings. As would be expected of a Region that is predominately rural in nature, the number of Decentralized C&E programs far surpassed the number of Centralized C&E units within the states of Connecticut, Maine, Massachusetts, New Hampshire and Vermont. There were some C&E programs that had been developed along the lines of a Mixed C&E Model, with these programs typically having a core staff of one or two individuals but relying heavily on staff from other center programs to provide C&E services.

As might be expected, the larger the size of the community mental health center, the greater the likelihood of a Centralized C&E Model. Historically, the primary purpose of the community mental health center has been the provision of direct clinical services. As such, it appears that it is only after clinical services have been developed and are meeting community needs that C&E programs begin to receive attention. This prioritization of clinical over consultative services cannot be overlooked in planning the organizational structure of the C&E program, since it is not unusual that allocated C&E time will be transformed into clinical service time during periods of high demand for treatment.

PROGRAM MODELS

The Centralized, Decentralized and Mixed organizational models for Consultation and Education will now be discussed in greater detail, with particular attention being given to the components of

— C&E Program Leadership
— C&E Program Planning, Delivery and Evaluation
— C&E Program Staffing and Financial support

A comparison of organizational models is facilitated when the key aspects of the leadership, services and supports are thought of as existing along a continuum from strong to weak. The greater the degree to which key components fall at the strong end of the continuum, the more viable the organizational model.

The Centralized Model

Organizationally, the Centralized Consultation and Education Model is perhaps the strongest of the three models. The C&E program is designed as a self-contained unit with a full-time director and full-time staff. In both belief and practice, the orientation of C&E staff is that of promoting positive mental health practices on the part of individuals, caregivers and organizational systems. The *vehicles* for attaining desired goals are the methods of consultation and education. The purpose of services is the prevention of emotional problems or very early identification and intervention. This is frequently the focus of C&E services targeted for children. The Centralized C&E Model offers strong opportunity for program identity on the part of staff with C&E staff referring to themselves as school consultants, early childhood consultants, industrial consultants or community educators rather than emphasizing that they are psychiatrists, psychologists, social workers or members of other disciplines. Optimally, the Centralized C&E program is elevated to the same organizational status as other clinical programs of the center, with the Director of Consultation and Education having authority and responsibility equal to that of the directors of various clinical programs. Given this level of authority and responsibility, the Director of C&E has immediate and equal access to the center director and an equal level of participation on the center's senior management team. For this to occur, the

Director of C&E must be full time. This individual is, in effect, the cornerstone of the C&E program, and the orientation, goals and objectives of the program itself will reflect the beliefs and attitudes of the C&E Director. The director has full authority and responsibility for all aspects of the C&E program and is also responsible for working closely with the directors of clinical services to facilitate a meaningful integration of C&E with other services offered by the center. The Director of C&E is also the individual upon whose shoulders rests the responsibility for the program's financial solvency and stability. This issue of financial responsibility cannot be taken lightly or relegated to a secondary position, as inadequate program funding is one of the major threats to the health and vitality of the C&E program. Where leadership is concerned, recruitment and selection of the Director of Consultation and Education must be undertaken carefully.

The areas of planning, delivery and evaluation of C&E services are a strength of the Centralized Model. A wealth of information exists on participatory decision making with benefits being that staff who are involved in planning and decisions are more highly motivated to follow through on planned approaches and to implement decisions in which they have felt a part. The Centralized Model facilitates C&E staff participation. Staff identify with and have a commitment to the C&E program, thus feeling involved in the functions of planning, service delivery and evaluation. Under the leadership of the C&E Director, and with the active participation of staff, a meaningful planned approach to Consultation and Education can occur, with the result being a clear definition of program goals, objectives, purposes and priorities.

Developing staffing and financial resources is another strength of the Centralized Model. When a center has made a decision to develop a Centralized C&E program, it has implicitly made a decision to finance the development of that program. Rarely do centers pursue a Centralized Model without an examination of the financial requirements of such a model. Initial C&E program funding is frequently acquired through some form of grant mechanism. However, grants are time limited. Since the Centralized Model is likely to be the most expensive of the three models, it is incumbent upon the C&E Director and staff actively to seek sources of continuing financial support during the period of seed money years. If there is a critical failing of C&E programs it is the instance of newly developed programs feeling too secure with their grant support and devoting inadequate attention to the future ramifications of the time-limited nature of grant support. Again, the Centralized Model can facilitate the pursuit of alternative funding resources. Staff themselves can become actively engaged in the development of contracts for services as, indeed, their own staff positions and livelihood are directly related to the maintenance of financial solvency of the C&E program.

Where C&E program staffing is concerned, the Centralized Model offers many advantages. It incorporates the concept of a full-time director who, given the necessary levels of authority, access to the center director and participation on the center's management team, can advocate for and protect the interests of the C&E program. Moreover, the staff of the C&E program do not have time commitments to any other program than their own. One of the frequently cited impediments to an effective C&E program is the siphoning off of C&E time during peak periods of demand for direct treatment services. The Centralized Model enables the C&E Director to retain control over the use of C&E staff time. Siphoning off can either be resisted completely or the C&E Director can agree to a limited reallocation of some time to address a centerwide concern. Thus, the Centralized Model possesses both the necessary flexibility and resistance to insure that C&E staff time is allocated to the primary mission of the program, that being the delivery of consultation and/or education services.

The Centralized C&E Model offers many strengths, but it also has weaknesses. The Centralized C&E program can become isolated from other programs in the center. If the Centralized C&E program has few staff, there may be a limited breadth of specialty skills. If the model does not maintain its flexibility, there may be skilled staff within clinical programs of the center who have an interest in providing limited consultation or education services but whose capabilities are not used because of too rigid program boundaries. Not to be overlooked is the perception of the C&E program by staff of clinical programs of the center. It is not uncommon for clinical staff to perceive C&E staff as having an easy

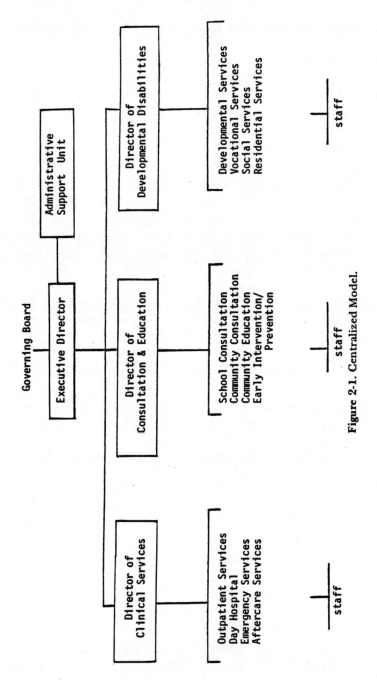

Figure 2-1. Centralized Model.

job compared to their own. Consultation or education roles can be readily misunderstood, perceived as easily implemented and as more fun than work. Often it is only when clinical staff themselves become involved in consultation activities and experience the resistance or frustrations often associated with attempts to function within an external system that they come to better understand and respect the difficult roles of C&E staff. In some ways it is understandable how misperceptions can occur. While clinical staff are office bound, C&E staff spend the majority of their time in the community. C&E staff often have diversity in their role and function. Clinical staff, by comparison, frequently feel tied to the same routine of seeing clients, one after the other, day after day. Over time, resentment can build. Unless it is confronted, the necessary relationships and linkages between C&E and other programs of the center can become undermined.

The Decentralized Model

The Decentralized Model for Consultation and Education is a design that incorporates a C&E Director or Coordinator, but without any full-time C&E staff. Instead, consultation and education services are provided by staff whose primary identity is with other programs of the center. The staff are *attached* to the Decentralized C&E program and devote a specifically allocated amount of time to C&E activities. The Decentralized Model is, therefore, sometimes referred to as the Percentage-Of-Time Model. The Decentralized Model, while perhaps less integrated than the Centralized Model, can still be a viable model for the delivery of C&E services given certain conditions. The model becomes viable when
  - the leadership of the C&E program is invested in a full-time director or coordinator and when that individual carries the necessary levels of program authority, responsibility, status and access to the center director.
  - the attached C&E staff devote a substantial percentage of their time to consultation and education activities, preferrably within the range of 40 percent to 60 percent, thereby facilitating at least a partial identity as C&E staff.

The Decentralized Model can quickly lose its effectiveness when leadership becomes invested in a part-time coordinator who, in reality, has little programmatic authority. Similarly, the Decentralized Model becomes less effective when staff attached to the C&E program spend only 5 percent or 10 percent of their time within the C&E program. These characteristics of a weak Decentralized program reflect a low priority for Consultation and Education within the mental health center and are, at best, a token effort with sparse recognition of the potential value and impact of C&E services. A weak Decentralized program is bound to fail. Leadership of any program can rarely be effectively provided on a part-time basis. This is particularly the case since the C&E Director or Coordinator will usually devote some time to the actual delivery of C&E services as part of the role. Part-time leadership allows insufficient time for the functions of planning, program development, evaluation of services, community liaison or the identification of alternative sources of financial support. When attached C&E staff spend a limited percentage of their time within the C&E program, this time is typically devoted to the actual delivery of consultation or education services. Resultantly, these staff too have insufficient time to participate meaningfully in planning or discussion of the goals and objectives of the C&E program or the charting of its future course. Support time *is* crucial, for without it the C&E program cannot possibly develop new programmatic efforts or expansions. A weak Decentralized Model reflects, at best, a limited commitment in both attitude and financial resources on the part of the center. Given this situation, a weak Decentralized C&E program will consistently be a low priority program for the center and a program first to be curtailed or eliminated in the face of financial crisis.

The Decentralized Model can be an effective model for C&E program development, and indeed, it is a model frequently used by rural mental health centers or centers of smaller size. Effective Decentralized programs have as their cornerstone a director or coordinator who devotes full time to the C&E program. Although this individual will not be directly hiring a full-time C&E staff, it is necessary that the C&E Director or Coordinator have significant input in the selection of staff from other programs who will also become part of the C&E staff. Optimally, the selection preferences of the C&E Director or Coordinator should be respected. Since a

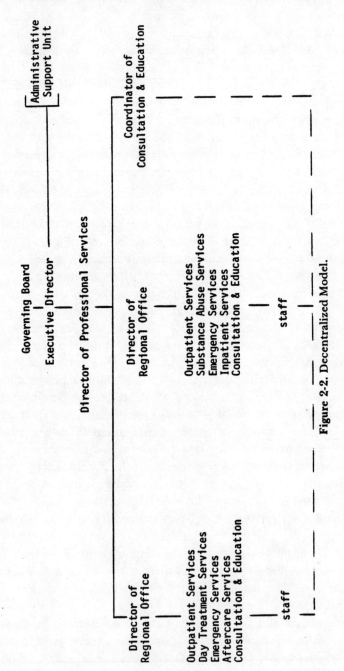

Figure 2-2. Decentralized Model.

great deal of networking with other center programs is required by the Decentralized Model, the actual time the C&E leader devotes to the delivery of consultation or education services should not be excessive. Inherent in the choice of a Decentralized Model is a nagging question about the degree to which a real commitment to C&E exists on the part of the center director and governing board. As such, the C&E Director or Coordinator will have to devote substantial time to the development of financial support for the program, since the C&E program itself could be considered to be an at-risk program.

Within the Decentralized Model, characteristics of planning, delivery and evaluation of services and the characteristic of staffing become interdependent. As has been previously stated, the Decentralized Model is more effective when fewer staff devote a greater percentage of their time to C&E activities as compared to a larger number of staff each devoting very little time. An interesting phenomenon that occurs around this issue of staff time is that staff themselves tend to affiliate with the program in which they spend a majority of their time. At a point where a given staff member spends approximately 60 percent time within a given program, there is a tendency to identify with that program area as well. Identity as a C&E *unit* can be formed within a Decentralized Model as long as the majority-time concept is recognized. To furthur clarify the manner in which a unit concept can be developed within a Decentralized Model, let us explore a hypothetical example.

Let us assume that a small rural community mental health center with a staff of twenty-five individuals wishes to explore the development of a Consultation and Education program. Let us also assume that the center director and the governing board have made a reasonable commitment to C&E by hiring a full-time coordinator to provide leadership for the newly developing program. Due to the center's size and a limited level of initial financial support, the center has decided that it can afford to hire the C&E Coordinator but it cannot afford to hire a distinct C&E staff. Therefore, the Decentralized model is adopted to allow for the reallocation of existing staff to the new C&E program. Initially, it is proposed that each of the twenty-five staff devote 10 percent of their time to Consultation and Education, totaling an equivalent of 2.5 staff positions. The newly hired C&E Coordinator, aware of the rule of majority-time, discusses this concept at a meeting of the center's senior management team. Since the C&E Coordinator has also met briefly with each of the twenty-five staff of the center, there is an awareness that not all staff have an interest in Consultation and Education but that four or five staff have a very strong interest and also have some prior experience providing consultation. Based upon this information, the C&E Coordinator offers the alternative proposal that instead of twenty-five staff devoting 10 percent time each to C&E activities, four staff with strong interest in C&E would each allocate 60 percent time to the new C&E program. The new majority-time proposal results in the same full-time staff equivalent as had been originally defined. Should the new proposal be accepted, the C&E Coordinator would have built a modified Centralized program within a Decentralized Model. Since the four individuals selected for the C&E program would spend the majority of their time within the C&E program, it is likely that these staff members would become identified as C&E staff, even though they retain a part-time clinical role.

Use of the majority-time approach does decrease the level of consultation or education services that can be delivered. This is because some time will be allocated to support activities such as program meetings, planning efforts and discussions of goals and objectives. Initially, it is more important for newly developing programs to build a sense of program identity among staff and to establish a solid planning base from which high quality services can be delivered than to minimize planning time in favor of service delivery.

The strength of a Decentralized Model for Consultation and Education is dependent upon the degree to which the Decentralized Model can approach a Centralized concept. The incorporation of the majority-time concept lends strength to the Decentralized Model and serves to build a program identity and facilitate the development of overall plans and objectives for the C&E program. The C&E Coordinator is better able to protect the C&E staff time from intrusion from other programs and, at the same time, maintain a link between clinical programs and C&E through staff also participating in clinical work. A greater likelihood exists for coordination among a smaller number of C&E staff, and given this smaller number, accountability is enhanced. Admittedly, there are limitations to having a smaller staff. A narrower range of expertise is represented among fewer C&E staff as opposed to the broader range of expertise that would exist among a greater complement of staff. Moreover, it is possible that there will be more community requests for consultation or education services than can be reasonably provided by a smaller staff.

Although equal in full time equivalent staff, the movement toward a more Centralized Model enhances the visibility of the Consultation and Education program. If the center's initial commitment to C&E is tenuous, this greater visibility may become a drawback. If, on the other hand, a genuine commitment to C&E services exists on the part of the center, then the C&E program would likely reap the benefits of high visibility.

The Decentralized Model can vary greatly in its organizational implementation and can be a model of strength or weakness. The model itself is neither inherently good nor bad, but it is rather the manner in which the model becomes translated into organizational existence that will have a significant impact upon Consultation and Education's future successes.

The Mixed Model

The Mixed Model is simply a blend of the Centralized and Decentralized Models previously described. The Mixed Model can evolve from a Decentralized approach or it can be the result of a Centralized C&E program having additional part-time staff attached to it. These part-time staff might join the C&E program for the purposes of meeting a very specific need that has been identified within the community. Let us briefly trace the development of a Mixed Model, first as a progression from a Decentralized Model and then as an adaptation of a small Centralized Model approach.

In tracing the progression of a Consultation and Education program from a Decentralized to a Mixed Model, let us recall the example of the small community mental health center discussed earlier in the chapter. We recall that initially the center's C&E program consisted of a full-time Coordinator and four C&E staff, each of which spent approximately 60 percent time within the C&E program. In charting the example, let us also assume that two of the C&E staff devoted 60 percent of their time to providing consultation services to local schools within the catchment area. The progression from Decentralized to a Mixed Model might be as follows:

As a result of satisfaction with a high quality service, the schools have decided to increase their contract for services. The new level of request for service will require an additional full-time individual. The Coordinator of C&E considers a number of possibilities to meet the new request for service:

1. To employ a full-time school consultant while maintaining the two former consultants at 60 percent time;
2. To increase the original school consultants' time to 100 percent time each and to employ another part-time school consultant at 20 percent time;
3. To maintain the original school consultants at 60 percent time each and to seek two additional school consultants at 50 percent time each.

The Coordinator of C&E explores the alternatives with the school consultants to assess their interest in expanding to full time, meets with the directors of clinical programs to assess the availability of additional staff time and expertise, and meets with the superintendent of schools to seek input on the possible alternatives. Based upon these contacts, it is concluded that the two existing consultants will expand to full-time work with the schools, and an additional individual will spend 20 percent time in school consultation. With implementation of this alternative the C&E program has moved from a Decentralized Model to a Mixed Model, now having a coordinator, two full-time school consultants and three part-time C&E staff (two of the original staff who continue to devote part time to C&E and an additional person who provides consultation to schools one day per week).

The Mixed C&E Model is typically of this composition, incorporating a small core staff who spend full time in the C&E program and a number of part-time staff who spend a percentage of time within C&E and a percentage of time within other programs of the center.

The Mixed C&E Model can also evolve from a Centralized Model. Let us consider a Centralized C&E unit consisting of full-time director and perhaps four or five full-time staff. Let us also assume that consultation or training for business and industry is identified as a desired focus of the C&E unit. The progression from Centralized to Mixed Models might be as follows:

The mental health center is approached by a local industry to discuss possibilities of providing consultation for management staff and to help in the development of a troubled employees program. In exploring this request, it becomes apparent that two areas of expertise are required to meet the need: expertise in alcohol abuse and in motivating troubled employees to seek assistance, and expertise in management consultation. In identifying two individuals to fulfill the role of consultants with industry, the C&E program has progressed from a Centralized Model to a Mixed Model, now incorporating a small core staff of full-time consultants as well as two part-time C&E staff to provide consultation to industry.

For purposes of clarification, it is important to note that the requirements of a Mixed Model include a blend of full-time and part-time C&E staff with full-time staff being limited in number. A Centralized C&E unit of a large community mental health center, which might incorporate fifteen to twenty full-time staff and only one or two part-time staff, would still be considered to be a Centralized Model rather than a Mixed Model. A requirement of the Mixed Model is that part-time staff providing C&E services be generally comparable in number with full-time staff. For many, this may seem like nitpicking about definitions, but since definitions are notoriously vague within the arena of Consultation and Education, efforts to become more explicit should be undertaken so as to create greater commonality and understanding about terms.

The Mixed Model shares many of the strengths and weaknesses of the Centralized and Decentralized Models. The cornerstone of the Mixed model is also a full-time director or coordinator with all of the authority, responsibility and access necessary to fulfill the role effectively. Although the full-time staff of the Mixed Model lends strength to the C&E program's capabilities for planning, evaluation of services and financial resource development,

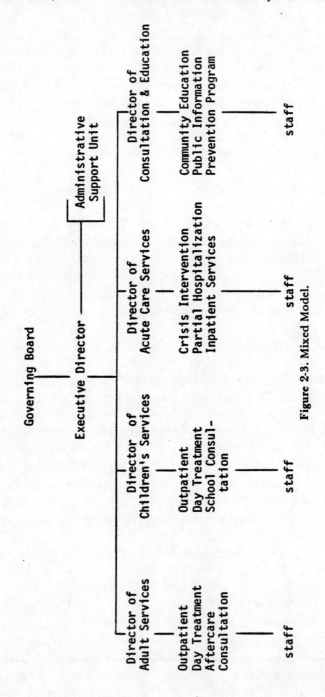

Figure 2-3. Mixed Model.

the Mixed Model also carries the weakness of some staff devoting small percentages of their time to C&E activities. It is often difficult for these individuals to participate actively in planning of the C&E program, with the result that they may feel less part of the C&E program than do the full-time staff. Since these part-time individuals are frequently piloting a new area of involvement, absence of their participation in planning meetings can frequently be a major loss to the C&E program. It is important, therefore, that the C&E leadership keep these individuals abreast of program directions and seek feedback on the potentialities and pitfalls of the new venture they are undertaking. If the Mixed Model is attained as a result of expansion from a Decentralized Model, this could be considered to be a significant step in the development of the C&E program, a step that reflects a stronger commitment to C&E on the part of the center. If, on the other hand, additional requests for C&E services lead simply to a further expansion of a Decentralized Model, without movement toward a full-time C&E staff, it is likely that levels of commitment and priority of C&E within the center have not changed.

Ad Hoc Approaches to Consultation and Education

Each of the three models for Consultation and Education previously outlined have the potential for delivering planned, directed and focused C&E activities. However, an approach to C&E services that is sorely lacking in those characteristics is sometimes called the Ad Hoc approach. Ad Hoc C&E services are essentially an effort on the part of some staff to provide C&E services based upon their own interest but without any formalized C&E structure. Ad Hoc C&E services almost always·develop in the face of substantial resistance to the implementation of a systematic approach to Consultation and Education. In some cases, an Ad Hoc consultation might receive sanction because it would be near political suicide for the center not to meet a given request. Maintaining the image of the center, rather than addressing the needs of the consultee, is a primary emphasis. The Ad Hoc approach to C&E services cannot by any stretch of the imagination be considered to be a model approach.

There are individuals who will argue that an Ad Hoc consultation is better than no consultation at all, but such a rationale must be seriously questioned. The existence of an Ad Hoc approach to C&E services can, in and of itself, be a major impediment to the development of a meaningful Consultation and Education program. If nothing else it offers grounds, although minimal, for the argument that the center is already providing C&E services, and therefore there is no reason to adopt an alternative model. Since change by its very nature creates imbalance in the status quo, it is frequently difficult to progress from an Ad Hoc approach to a meaningful model approach. Given this consideration, it may be preferable to delay the development of Consultation and Education should the initiation of such a program meet with substantial resistance. If C&E is unable to be developed in a meaningful fashion, it is better that the service not exist at all than exist in a manner that will likely fail to deliver the quality and range of services that the community would come to expect.

A LOOK TOWARD THE FUTURE

The Integrated Community Service Model

Any discussion of organizational structures would be incomplete without a recognition of the impending state and federal forces that will shape community mental health in the near future, and with it Consultation and Education. To borrow a descriptor from education, the trend in mental health services is "back to basics." The shift of responsibility for mental health services from the federal to state level, and a concurrent move toward block grant funding, have major ramifications for *community* mental health. Historically, state departments of mental health have identified the care of the chronic mentally ill as *the* priority of state funding. In years gone by, the institution was the primary mechanism of care. Today, as a result of deinstitutionalization, community mental health center precare and aftercare programs are the main providers of services, with services being supported by the state. The drain of state monies to provide care to a sizable mentally ill population within the community is substantial. It is a fiscal reality that few dollars remain to finance other services.

Nationally, the trend is toward a reduction of social service expenditures. Indeed, even some states have reached their own fiscal crises; reference California's Proposition 13 and Massachusetts's Proposition 2½. The time may soon arrive when state and federal support of even the chronic mentally ill population becomes jeopardized. Simply stated, the *community* will no longer be emphasized as part of community mental health.

For Consultation and Education, the implications are awesome. Those C&E programs whose main emphasis is the support of chronic care, through services such as consultation to community care homes or institutions, carry potential for future state support of C&E services. However, those C&E programs or services directed toward the general community will need to fend for themselves. The future outlook for Consultation and Education is less than positive, and it would be understandable for C&E to adopt a Chicken Little posture, proclaim that "the sky is falling," and wait for it to crash down upon us. However, C&E has always faced struggles, and this is but another problem that confronts it. Those C&E programs which recognize and accept the challenge will survive. There appear to be two options: (1) for C&E to redirect its philosophy and service priorities toward the support of the chronic mentally ill; or (2) for C&E to attempt to maintain its broad community focus in the face of difficult circumstances and funding restraints. Either avenue can lead to survival. Each is a pro-active effort to address a critical issue. Both are compromises, the former compromising philosophy over dollars, the latter dollars over philosophy. C&E programs have always been idiosyncratic to their own community mental health centers (Yolles, 1977), and again this will be so. As overall CMHC priorities go, so too must go C&E.

For those CMHCs whose executive director and governing board sanction a retention of a broad community service despite losses of funding, the Integrated Community Service Model offers a viable approach. It is interesting to note that C&E is not alone in its struggle for survival. Community *outpatient* services also face serious reductions in state and federal funds. Thus, it is both C&E *and* clinical staff who face the dilemmas of service and funding that accompany the choice of community versus chronic populations. C&E and clinical staff who previously vied against one another now find themselves on the same side of the funding fence — the outside. Together, they represent the core of true *community* services. As allies, they have the potential to retain the community services of community mental health.

The Integrated Model

The Integrated Community Service is perhaps more a concept than a model, as the word *model* connotes an approach that has withstood the test of time and has demonstrated its value and validity. It is a rare CMHC, indeed, that has a proven and time-tested Integrated Community Service. There are a few centers that have adopted this approach and are pioneering the concept, and it is these centers which have created *corporate configurations* consisting of multiple non-profit entities under the auspices of the overall CMHC governing board.

The Integrated Community Service is, perhaps, the ultimate Mixed Model. No longer one that limits its functions to C&E, it entails a blend of all community services — both direct and indirect. Organizationally, there is a melding of traditional outpatient and C&E services under a unified leadership and philosophy. The integrated service has a single purpose: to maintain service to the general public. It represents the original concept of community mental health. The staff and leadership of the Integrated Service are typically well credentialed and seasoned professionals who are entrepreneurial in their own right. Each of these qualities is important, as we will see when financial aspects of the Integrated Model are discussed. Programmatic leadership can come from more than one individual, but the integration of services and fiscal responsibilities is invested in the group's most capable manager. Whether the leadership of the Integrated Model possesses a C&E or clinical background does not matter, since C&E and clinical entities no longer compete against one another. The model is one in which C&E and clinical services become interrelated and interdependent. C&E services provide the necessary level of community visibility through educational programs or linkage with consultee agencies, while clinical services act as a point of referral for the C&E staff. An overall systems approach integrates C&E with clinical so that

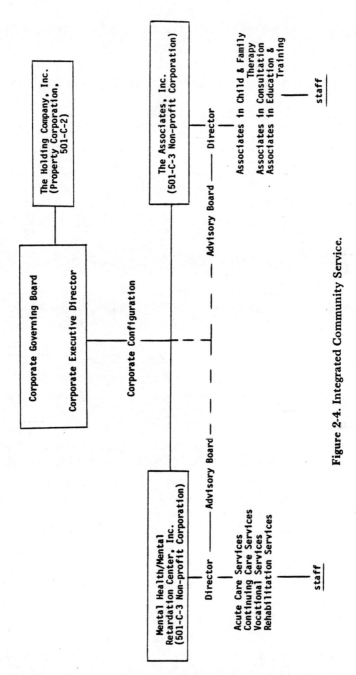

Figure 2-4. Integrated Community Service.

therapists and consultants work hand in hand to achieve a maximum benefit for the individual client or family. The model offers the potential for a level of integration that rarely exists today among C&E and clinical programs in community mental health centers.

Organizationally, there is flexibility in staff service roles. Staff devote full time to C&E, full time to clinical services, or provide a combination of both. The siphoning off of staff time from C&E to clinical (even clinical to C&E) is a moot point since all staff work under performance contracts that identify specific functions and service expectations. Staff salary is linked directly to these performance contracts, the result being that staff carry responsibility for their own livelihood. Preferrably, there is a single locale where the Integrated Community Service is located, another bond even if a symbolic one of the integration of C&E and clinical. Should the Community Service be an entity of a broader corporate configuration, the ties to the parent CMHC might be kept at a low level of visibility. This is particularly true if the CMHC itself has adopted a major chronic care emphasis that might negatively carry over to the Community Service. In such cases, the Integrated Community Service might even have its own name, one that connotes its community orientation, affiliate status, or associate grouping.

Financing of the Integrated Model involves a blend of service contracts, fees for service and staff entrepreneurial skill. Active effort is given to contracts for services, whether they are contracts for consultation or service agreements with business and industry for prepaid counseling/therapy for employees in need. The concept of fee for service pervades the fiscal approach of an Integrated Model, regardless of whether services are clinical, consultative or educational. Clinical services are still able to be provided to clients of varying income levels, but perhaps in a more limited way. As example, clinical services might be provided under a client matrix that designates a certain number of clients who are able to be served at each fee level and that yields an average moderate fee level of income that is consistently derived from clinical services. Adjusting the matrix in turn varies the level of client fee income, whether this is upward or downward. Should demand for clinical services be high, then multiple waiting lists are created and managed. Treatment itself is predominately short term, although long-term therapy can be provided to a limited degree based upon the client matrix.

Consultation and Education also carry fees for service. Free services are rarely, if ever, provided. Fees for C&E services are established at a level that reimburses the cost of delivering the service. When opportunities present themselves, C&E services are contracted back to the parent CMHC as, for example, a contract under which the Integrated Service develops a training program for CMHC staff who provide service to chronic populations.

Financial support is also attained through the CMHC itself allocating community monies such as those from a local United Way campaign to the community service. This CMHC subsidy helps to support educational or clinical services to individuals who otherwise could not afford to take advantage of such services. Grants, when available, round out the financial picture.

At first glance, the Integrated Community Service Model may seem akin to a private practice approach, but it is not. The Model seeks to sustain the primary intent embodied in the original CMHC legislation. Services to individuals of all income levels are maintained, even if in matrix form, while the full range of services from prevention through clinical intervention is offered to the community. What the model *does* is integrate that range of educational, consultative and clinical services in a meaningful manner.

For many years, C&E has expended energy protecting itself from the intrusion of clinical services. It is energy that C&E can no longer afford to misdirect toward internal CMHC issues. Instead, effort is needed elsewhere if both C&E and outpatient services are to face the challenge of their own survival. Since it is common knowledge that financial crises tend to reduce program boundaries that otherwise seem rigid and impenetrable, the present-day funding curtailments from a state and federal level bring with them an interesting opportunity for growth. The Integrated Community Service represents this direction of growth. It is an organizational model that is responsive to changes in federal and state priorities in services and funding, and it is one that retains a broad range of services to the general community. While the Integrated Community Service is a model for the future, it is also an approach that will be viewed by some as the demise of C&E. Ultimately, it is a matter of perspective, either presenting the challenge of a new beginning for C&E or sounding its death knell.

REFERENCES

1. Perlmutter, F. D. Consultation and Education in Rural Community Mental Health Centers. *Community Mental Health Journal*, 1979, *15*(1), 58-68.
2. Rabow, A. K., & Rabow, P. J. *Let's Not Re-Invent the Wheel.* Proceedings of the First Annual Region I Consultation and Education Conference, Killington, Vermont, October, 1978.
3. Yolles, S. F. A critical appraisal of community mental health services. In Serban (Ed.), *New Trends of Psychiatry in the Community.* Cambridge: Ballinger Press, 1977.

Chapter 3

STAFFING AND TRAINING
IN CONSULTATION AND EDUCATION

JOHN C. FREUND

NEARLY half of all Consultation and Education services provided by community mental health center staff are in the
form of case consultations delivered by clinicians functioning as
part-time staff of the C&E program. A smaller but growing proportion of consultation and education activities involves community consultation, education and training provided by educators and paraprofessionals who represent a variety of back-
grounds. Staffing is, indeed, a critical area for the C&E program.
This chapter will focus on the development of clinicians as consultants and will also address staffing and training issues involved
in the growing use of educators and paraprofessionals for community consultation, education and training.

THE CLINICIAN AS CONSULTANT

Community mental health centers may effectively develop or
expand their Consultation and Education programs through the
use of clinical staff. With expertise in individual, group and family
treatment skills, clinicians may well be the most appropriate individuals to enter into consultation relationships with community
agencies and institutions. The goals of such consultation are frequently the creation of linkages between helping agents and the
provision of a teaching/learning forum for caregivers in the community. For many clinicians, bridging the gap between clinical

and consultation approaches involves an exploration of alternative views of the helping process. Clinicians are familiar with the one-to-one dyad of psychotherapy. Within their new role of consultant, trainer or agency-to-agency liaison, however, clinicians must become aware of the significant increase in potential for clinical impact, not to mention their unsettling awareness that therapeutic impact occurs indirectly through the improvement of the quality of auxiliary helping services on the part of community caregivers. Thus, the following discussion of the clinician-consultant role involves consideration of a systems perspective of the helping process, the implications of structure and setting on the consultant's role, internal and external supports, personal and professional identity issues, and a discussion of the range of functions of the clinician-consultant.

The Geometric Effect of C&E Services

Clinician services usually suggest an arithmetic approach to helping, either one by one, one by couple, one by group, or one by family. Clinician-consultants have the opportunity to have an impact upon the immediate client via case consultation and also to influence the treatment of future clients of the consultee agency. Within a training or program consultation role, the opportunities for exponential impact are even greater. Thus, the effect becomes geometric. To cite an example, consultation concerning the psychological adjustment of one senior citizen to a nursing home directly affects that senior citizen and can have some limited effects upon future clients. Expansion of the focus of consultation to the broader problem of senior citizens' entry into nursing homes presents a remarkably more powerful potential for impact, encompassing perhaps even the question of the mental health of the community. It is important to recognize that clinical skills employed to assist the individual and his/her family are a vital ingredient in assisting a nursing home to facilitate client entry.

The role of the clinician-consultant requires a multidimensional view of human behavior. A clinician concerned about an individual senior citizen attends primarily to psychological, physical, cognitive and social dimensions of the individual's experience. The clinician-consultant attends to these factors and many others.

Clinician-consultants are concerned about individuals within environments, as defined by a host of setting, staffing, legal, economic and other variables. The focus becomes one of concern for helping systems, their functioning and impact upon present and future clients. Systems entry, such as into nursing homes, might be viewed as an issue of psychological preparation of clients and their families, but it may also be an issue of staff schedules, staff training, or physical location of new residents.

Systems Impact

It is clearly unrealistic to expect the clinician-consultant to be able to deal effectively with the breadth of variables affecting complex helping systems. Meaningful impact requires a team effort and usually demands extensive collaboration, cooperation and support among community agencies and institutions. Ideally, the clinician-consultant can mobilize individuals and systems toward a broad spectrum approach to helping. The consultant can, in the process, stimulate dialogue and action that promote the clarification of community agencies' areas of responsibility.

The clinician-consultant will have contact with a wide variety of helpers, agencies and institutions. Through these efforts, communication networks can be built to improve service delivery substantially. The mythical senior citizen of our example benefits when local physicians, physical therapists, meal site counselors, transportation people, nurses and the many others involved in the lives of senior citizens help rather than struggle with one another as they understand and effectively coordinate their mandates and methods of functioning.

The clinician-consultant carries the potential to have an impact upon clients, caregivers and human service delivery systems. The possibilities are both exciting and challenging: exciting in the opportunity for meaningful impact; challenging inasmuch as opportunities for impact also vary directly with the complexity of the problems, the difficulty of the consulting issues, the effects of the current goals and programs of the mental health center and the external needs of service systems as they relate to the cultural and social processes of the community at large.

The Clinician-Consultant Role

The repertoire of roles available to the clinician-consultant will be determined by the interplay of a number of factors. Considerations must be given to the breadth of clinical and community skills of the consultant, the extent of supervisory and support personnel available to the consultant, the image of the mental health center among community caregivers, and the Consultation and Education structure established for the delivery of services. The consultant must also be cognizant of the expertise and level of skills among other human service providers external to the mental health center. The following presents a range of potential roles of the clinician-consultant, presented in rank order from most clinical and least community involved to least clinical and most community involved:

Clinician In-house: The clinician strictly provides individual, group and family treatment within one of the many traditional models of therapy. Services are office based within the mental health center, clinic or hospital. The clinician responds to the expressed emotional and social needs and concerns of patients or clients.

Clinician In-community: The clinician functions in much the same way as the clinician in-house except that therapeutic services are delivered within a community setting, such as a department of probation, nursing home, school or other social service agency. The clinician has more extensive contact with the referring agent, and the clients may not view themselves as paying for the service. Clinicians within this role frequently specialize in a particular client population. Clinical work in a community setting can provide an excellent opportunity for clinicians to experience the realities of helping from the perspective of other community caregivers. This knowledge of community caregivers' functions, and of the conditions under which they work, lays the groundwork for escalation to a more complex role of clinician as consultant.

Clinician As Consultant: The clinician-consultant role is an outgrowth of the two strains of clinical and community approaches previously described. The clinician-consultant provides a range of services, including case consultation, staff consultation, third party negotiation, agency-to-agency linkage, or support of other helping staff. Central to all of these roles is the application of clinical skills, in divergent settings, within a secondary helping role. The critical element is that the clinician-consultant no longer fulfills the role of direct helper but, instead, becomes a helper to other helpers. The overall focus of the clinician-consultant remains largely client outcome, and the emphasis of the role is still somewhat clinician over consultant.

Consultant As Trainer: In this role, the consultant sheds the primary identification as a clinician in favor of functioning as a trainer or teacher. Clinical skills are taught, and the prime concern is the enhancement of skills or knowledge on the part of other caregivers. Consultant as trainer focuses on the impact of training activities upon the long- and short-term functioning of community caregivers within the context of their current agency mandate. Training, then, is not merely for the sake of knowledge and skill development but relates directly to the current functioning and future development of the consultee agency.

Consultant As Systems Change Agent: The systems change agent functions within or across helping systems with a goal of complete or partial restructuring of those systems. As an organizational development consultant, systems consultant, or mental health/human relations consultant, the practitioner seeks to alter such factors as case load, supervision, subunit relations, staffing or other conditions that impede the most effective delivery of services for a given agency. The systems consultant seeks to link agencies, clarify roles in the community, or assist in resolving interagency differences. It is within the Systems Change Agent role that the consultant has the clearly articulated goal of effecting change, much as a clinician seeks to effect change when confronted with traditional clinical client problems.

Community Consultant/Organizer: A community organization role borders on the political and is the farthest removed from traditional clinical functioning. The community consultant seeks to organize the community, or subsets of it, to have a positive impact upon the collective mental health. The community consultant establishes a network among members of the community, individuals who are in no way identified as clients or patients. This consultant is a community systems change agent, as opposed to a human service delivery systems change agent. The clinician consultant model comes full circle with this role, as the clinician in-house and the community consultant/organizer have the most direct contact with the community at large.

These brief descriptions of potential roles for the clinician considering a consultant's role clearly do not do justice to the complexity involved. The following discussion, therefore, will expand upon the many external, internal (to the mental health center) and personal issues that affect the emerging consultant. Factors such as these affect consultants in more extensive and potent ways as those individuals extend themselves farther and farther from the traditional mental health clinical role.

CRITICAL ISSUES OF THE CONSULTANT ROLE

External Factors

As a consultant working in the community, an individual assumes an agency representative role to a significantly enlarged degree. The community's view of mental health professionals, and even a particular agency's competence, is directly linked to the behavior and performance of the consultant. For many clinicians, whose primary allegiance has been to a professional discipline or school of therapy, the identification as a representative of the mental health center may have troublesome implications. Thus, the issue of allegiance or loyalty arises. Centers, hospitals and clinics are always embroiled to some degree in community or regional politics of service delivery and funding. Traditional clinicians are usually sheltered from such turmoil. Clinician-consultants, on the other hand, often walk the tightrope of mixed allegiances to client, to consultee agency, to profession and to agency as employer. The transition from client focus to conflictual allegiance between consultee and employer agency requires a major personal, behavioral and conceptual shift. In fact, it is not unknown for a consultant to assist a consultee agency to negotiate more effectively a difficult relationship with the consultant's own agency.

A second external factor to consider is the mental health center's historical relationship with community agencies and institutions and the posture or position of the mental health center vis-à-vis community care-giving agencies. Consultee staff and agencies will only use consultation or implement a consultant's recommendations to the extent that the mental health center has cooperated with the consultee agency in providing support and services to their particular troubled or disturbed population. The question becomes "Is the mental health center willing to be of assistance if a consultee's effort to provide an expanded or revised helping role fails?" Clearly, the external posture of the community mental health center must coincide with its ability to deliver the backup services represented by its verbal posture. This presents a dramatic departure from traditional clinicians' primary reliance upon themselves and possibly a few colleagues, as the consultant relies heavily upon the community mental health center as a service system.

A third external consideration is the reality of mandates, restraints and sanctions that affect the functioning of staff of community agencies and institutions. Those mandates often incorporate vastly different assumptions about behavior and service delivery. The five major systems, education, health, social service, mental health and criminal justice, have all experienced considerably different historical development and represent sometimes radically different traditions of practice. Consultants need to be aware of and respect the limits for change presented by agency history, tradition and mandates, for failure to attend to such structural realities sets the consultant up to appear naive and undermines consultee staff motivation. Above all, the consultant must avoid the arrogance that so many insensitive clinicians have fallen prey to in their initial attempts at helping consultees.

Concern for the quality of the interaction between consultant and consultee agency staff cannot be overemphasized. The consultant must be cautious not to intrude where assistance has not been requested, for resentment is possible because of implied inadequacy. Mental health center consultants invariably face the question of why staff of the mental health center always seek to function as consultants or trainers to community agencies but never use community agency staff in the capacity of consultants to the CMHC. It is a question well taken.

As a summary of concerns that stem from factors external to the community mental health center, the following should be highlighted: (1) that service delivery will be affected because clinicians will be involving others, possibly many others, in their work; (2) that a variety of new dimensions of functioning will emerge because, at some level, the consultant may be involved with clients of other agencies; (3) that consultants need to be cognizant of the dissonance that can occur between goals of training or consultation and the consultee agency case load or mandate; and, (4) that consultants must respond to the multiple variables flowing from their agency representative role.

Internal factors

Internal factors refer to conditions within the community mental health center that affect the viability of the clinician-consultant role. Such variables as the C&E program's structural organization, staffing pattern, funding and recordkeeping can either support or detract from an effective consultation posture. On a broader level, one must honestly assess the degree of understanding of and support for the mental health center fulfilling the role of consultant or trainer in the community.

A first internal factor to be considered is the C&E program's organizational structure within the community mental health center. While federal guidelines require a discrete Consultation and Education program, this mandate is adhered to more in form than substance. Clearly, the clinician-consultant will be most successful when functioning as part of a service unit that views its responsibility as the extension of skills and service into the community. General center organization and specifically access to center leaders can have a profound affect on the clinician-consultant role. The federal government anticipated this concern in requiring that Directors of Consultation and Education programs have clear lines of access to center directors who are likely to have extensive contact with leaders of other community agencies. Information flow between clinician-consultants and individuals in leadership positions is vital for the clinician-consultant to attain a broad understanding of interagency functioning.

The internal factor of professional discipline roles and values cannot be overlooked. Unfortunately, members of some disciplines feel they have a corner on particular aspects of the helping process. Except for the psychiatrist's control of medication and some aspects of neurophysiology, the remainder of clinician-consultant activities should be available to all mental health professionals regardless of discipline. For many years, community work and client care were the concern of social workers and to some extent public health nurses. Social psychiatry and community psychology, among other disciplines, are clearly considered to be Johnny-come-lately in some quarters. Realistically, the clinician-consultant, regardless of professional discipline, can become embroiled in community affairs that cannot possibly be adequately conceptualized. On the whole, however, the clinician-consultant's depth of knowledge in the area of human behavior does support venturing into the broader community system. To the extent that professional discipline conflicts prevail, cross-disciplinary work and nontraditional mental health service will need careful nurturance within professional's own groups.

The internal factors of time, funding, accountability and recordkeeping present themselves for review. It takes substantial preparation and planning time to be a clinician-consultant. Travel time alone eats significantly into the consultant's day. Preparation activities are essential for effective clinician-consultant functioning; thus, the center's time and accountability structures should give work credit for these functions. Strategies that include credit for preparation and appreciate reasonable levels of direct contact hours add support to the clinician-consultant's internal relations. Creating appropriate consultation records, similar in intent to clinical case records, facilitates support evaluation and monitoring efforts on the part of supervisors and administrators. A final internal factor affecting the clinician-consultant is staff relations. Traditional clinicial staff inevitably experience mixed emotions about clinician-consultants. On one hand, they may deprecate the "non-mental health," "indirect" nature of the clinician-consultant's work. On the other hand, this deprecation may reflect jealousy or resentment of the clinician-consultant's apparent freedom to move across the numerous traditional physical and functional boundaries of mental health service delivery. The support of staff of clinical programs may be cultivated if the clinician-consultant has an impact on their referral networks (especially if the clinician-consultant can help decrease levels of inappropriate referrals). The clinician-consultant's efforts to help community agencies and institutions to attend effectively to their clients may eventually endear them to traditional clinical staff. Maintaining staff relationships through participation in staffings and case conferences may also assist in the support of strong internal networks.

The description of internal factors affecting the clinician-consultant is not exhaustive. It does serve to highlight the critical concerns raised by many clinicians and consultants. One final issue remains. From an ethical perspective the question of "who is responsible for the clients affected by the clinician-consultant's work with consultee agencies and institutions?" must be addressed. This issue can raise important individual and personal issues for the clinician-consultant. As an interagency issue, the question of client responsibility must be resolved as a legal contractual matter between the mental health center and the consultee agency. As an issue in the emergence of the clinician-consultant, it is perhaps the most difficult personal factor to be resolved, as, from a consultation perspective, the consultee retains complete responsibility and control over client treatment. The consultant is but an advisor whose recommendations can be rejected by the consultee as readily as they can be accepted. The clinician-consultant's awareness of the ability to "influence" but not directly "control" client treatment can be a most difficult realization.

Personal Factors

The first of a number of personal issues for the clinician-consultant is the transition from the role of direct helper to that of a role of being secondary, consultant-to-helper. Combinations of personal dynamics and clinical training have frequently supported needs on the part of clinicians to have direct personal helping impact and to take responsibility for individual client outcomes. Direct clinical services, are, for many, an outgrowth of personal need structures. The prevention and geometric impact notions accompanying a consultant role challenge the individual to attend to a larger audience. While this seductive position is appealing, it can also be marred by linear and arithmetic faults destined to confuse and undermine the new role of the clinician-consultant.

Functioning as a clinician-consultant does not mean arithmetically more traditional helping services. Clinical treatments suggest a cause-effect, linear relationship between therapist-client behavior and outcome. The number of variables extant in the treatment setting are finite and, to some extent, under therapist and client control. Within the clinician-consultant role, effect is usually diluted. Situational variables, over which the clinician-consultant exercises little control, frequently intrude upon the consultation process to the point that consultees may or may not show significant changes in their own behavior or therapeutic approaches with clients.

In the same manner that a client experiences crisis because usual responses are dysfunctional in stressful situations, so too the clinician-consultant may face functional crisis because traditional training can be insufficient preparation for the challenges of consultation situations. Adaptation to and success in a clinician-consultant role require additional learning and some risk taking. Fortunately, many of the difficulties confronting the clinician-consultant are related to psychological realities that are familiar to traditional clinicians as a result of their therapeutic work with clients. First and foremost, clinician-consultants must have a high tolerance for ambiguity. Whereas in some clinical contexts it is the clinician who creates the ambiguity, within consultation it is the complex reality of the community that creates a lack of clarity. The impact of ambiguity on the clinician-consultant produces similar opportunities for choosing alternatives as are presented to clients by traditional clinicians. Clinician-consultants may respond to their own needs or they may struggle with consultee systems as they work toward productive resolution of situations.

The personal factor of need for successful outcome of consultation episodes can lead to frustration for the clinician-consultant. Consultee systems provide little direct feedback, and the outcome effects of consultation are often not readily apparent. This is

especially the case when a goal of consultation is creating awareness or facilitating productive discussion of systems issues rather
then direct treatment concerns. Related to this issue of outcome
is the nature of the clinician-consultant's visibility and vulnerability. As clinician-consultants struggle with methods to measure outcomes in traditional terms, they remain highly visible and vulnerable to criticism or attack from client, consultee or internal support systems. Direct clinical services are typically more protected
from observation and critique by colleagues and the community.
Conversely, systems issues raised in consultation may reverberate
far beyond consultation participants, particularly when hidden
agendas exist that are very different from those of the leaders
of the consultant and consultee agencies. Even the clinician-
consultant is not immune to this situation, as the consultant's
agenda may vary considerably from the goals and objectives of the
consultation itself. The realities of these discrepant agendas and
the high visibility of consultation work creates a level of vulnerability that the clinician-consultant must clearly recognize.

Clinician consultants frequently work on the boundaries of
human service systems. As the visibility-vulnerability issue suggests, clinician-consultants must carefully attend to the extent of
their involvement with both internal support units and with consultee systems. Sometimes the function of the clinician-consultant
is to facilitate interface between these and other systems. Person-
ally, this leaves the consultant very much betwixt and between,
constantly balancing personal, professional and contractual loyalties. Too strong an identification with the traditions of one profession, service or community group can readily interfere with the
consultant's effectiveness. Although the clinician's dilemma
around the level of involvement with clients is clearly analogous
to the consultant's concern, the clinical issue lacks the complexity
and insecurity that may arise in consultation.

To become a clinician-consultant, an individual must face the
personal issues of broadening one's identity as a helper. Factors
such as dealing with ambiguity, visibility, vulnerability, lack of
feedback and unmeasurable outcomes are ongoing issues for the
clinician-consultant and require a serious reexamination of both
the individual's personal dynamics and professional identity as a
helper.

STAFFING AND TRAINING FOR COMMUNITY
CONSULTATION AND EDUCATION

Now that considerable discussion has been given to the development of the clinician-consultant role, which is based upon sound clinical skills supported by the acquisition of consultation skills and the necessary awareness to function in divergent community settings, the focus will shift to issues involved in the training and selection of C&E staff who have not been grounded in clinical activity. While many of the same considerations concerning functioning in the community have an impact upon the work of community educators or trainers, these individuals are usually less burdened by the personal dynamics and personal-vocational concerns of the clinician-consultant. Lest the reader begin to believe that these Consultation and Education staff are without serious staffing and training concerns, careful examination should be given to the following catalogue of contentious issues.

Specialist Vs. Generalist Staff

Ideally community mental health centers, and Consultation and Education Programs in particular, are staffed by individuals who possess more than one area of expertise. The specialist, employed by a center to work exclusively with a single community agency or institution, usually develops a greater allegiance with the consultee or the specialty discipline than with the CMHC. Should a need for the specialty consultant cease to exist, or should funding be curtailed, there is rare support for a single-area specialist to continue with the center. Specialists in such areas as criminal justice, aging, health care or education can encounter considerable difficulty in identifying with the broader goals of community mental health. To cite a cliché, specialists with narrow allegiances or skill repertoires can miss the forest for the trees. This is not to say that specialists should not be employed by the CMHC.

There are benefits to a C&E program having some specialists on staff, and where community needs are substantial, specialists may be supported for extensive periods. Specialists in such areas as aging, school consultation, substance abuse or criminal justice, to name a few, may play a valuable, supportive role to clinical staff providing treatment services. Specialists are able to provide consultation, education and training for both staff of the CMHC and community caregivers. Within the consultation arena particularly, specialists are considerably more familiar with the subtleties of consultee systems and speak the language of the consultee as opposed to the jargon of human services. These specialists can help clinicians and community caregivers become aware of advancing developments within the specialized field and can facilitate the learning of alternative treatment approaches. Additionally, specialists can raise the consciousness of the community by offering educational presentations, courses, workshops and seminars relating to the area of specialization.

The arguments are inconclusive regarding specialist versus generalist staff selection. Community need situations will play a determining role in the CMHC's recruitment of specialist staff. Many of the problems inherent in the specialist model can be mitigated by thoughtful planning and organization. Yet, prudence suggests that Consultation and Education programs would do well to maintain an overall responsiveness based upon a cadre of well-trained generalists, with specialists or specialist teams being used as appropriate and feasible.

Clinical Vs. Educational Staff

Consultation and Education staff possessing a clinical background have the distinct advantage of sharing considerable history, training and approach with staff of other programs of the center. They are likely to be more positively perceived as part of the mental health endeavor and gain greater acceptance and support from treatment staff than would educationally trained individuals. Clinically trained C&E staff may also have the capability to deliver specific assistance around difficult consultee clients. This enhanced level of clinical assistance can serve as both an inroad and a building block for credibility, factors necessary to the development of future consultation, training or educational programs. These same clinically trained C&E staff may, however, encounter difficulty bridging the gap toward a more preventive or consultative approach to work with the community.

The use of educational staff underscores the C&E program's attempt to provide a variety of learning experiences for staffs of community caregiving agencies and for the community-at-large. Some clinically oriented staff are excellent teachers, but educationally oriented staff are far more "expert" in the process of creating effective learning environments. Assuming that the creation of receptivity to mental health education, training and consultation is at the very heart of consultation and education activities, then educational staff become a distinct asset. Moreover, educational staff most clearly emphasize a learning, growth-oriented perspective, rather than the restorative, rebuilding model of traditional clinicians.

A major drawback of educational staff is that they usually lack the clinical credentials and experience that allow them to "double" as staff for reimbursable treatment activities. Compensation for this potential funding impediment may well exist through educational staff's ability to design and implement fundable education and training programs for community agencies and institutions. Indeed, a point rarely examined by CMHC administrators is that C&E educational staff's delivery of community training courses or workshops may result in monthly income levels that would require a clinician multiple months to match based upon sliding fee scales. Although educators may have an initial disadvantage in establishing credibility for C&E training functions, those learning and training approaches, once implemented, are apt to have a more lasting impact on the community.

Optimally, a blend of clinical and educational staff is desirable within the Consultation and Education program; this integration can lead to a powerful team approach. Within the CMHC itself, the proportion of educational and clinical staff depends on the posture of the center and the goals and objectives of the C&E program. Well-established mental health centers, or those which are clearly community oriented, have less need to emphasize clinical credibility via the C&E program, as it is likely that community caregivers have been involved in consultation or training relationships over past years. CMHCs with newly developing C&E programs, or those which have historically represented a strong clinical as opposed to community orientation, would do well to develop clinically oriented C&E programs to expand upon their past clinical relationships with community agencies.

Professional Vs. Paraprofessional Staff

The literature is replete with information on the use and development of paraprofessional staff in community mental health. While it is accurate to say that paraprofessionals may extend the efforts of professional staff, it is also clear that paraprofessionals require considerable supervision and support. When the limits of paraprofessional functioning are clearly defined, and when appropriate training and supervision are provided, paraprofessional staff can be used effectively. Unfortunately, the more common use of paraprofessional staff occurs when a CMHC is short staffed and seeks to employ paraprofessionals in service roles that extend well beyond their boundaries of competence. The result of such practice can readily be disaster.

Paraprofessional roles need to be considered very carefully. Paraprofessionals may successfully fulfill the role of community liaison, provide information and referral, perform advocacy functions or teach concrete skills of daily living. Education and training roles that require significant background in human development, personality or psychopathology are better left to professionals. It is regrettable that paraprofessionals are often inappropriately used, such as a case of providing an individual with a script and set of techniques and expecting leadership of a parenting class. Use of paraprofessionals in this manner not only limits the breadth of opportunities that arise in many community education programs but also does a disservice to the paraprofessional staff person.

Use of Community Resources

The involvement of community resource persons in C&E education and training programs strongly supports connections among helping agents and agencies within the community. Many education and training topics readily lend themselves to interdisciplinary presentations. Programs for new parents, women approaching menopause, the aged and teachers may involve a variety of health, mental health, social service and educational personnel. Other topics such as family violence may suggest the cooperation of clergy, police, criminal justice, health, social services and mental health staff. The combinations and possibilities are extensive, with cosponsorship of educational programs serving to support the development of cohesive bonds among critical elements of the community caregiving system.

Use of community resource persons reduces the likelihood of mental health staff extending themselves beyond their areas of competence. An incidental benefit of coordinated educational presentations, such as that which might involve a physician, nurse, law enforcement officer and social worker, is that these individuals come to understand one another's role in the community of helpers. A C&E staff person may fulfill the role of moderator or may present a small portion of a program. In other instances, the C&E staff person may encourage and support another agency to assume leadership for a program.

CONCLUSION

Responsibilities for staff selection and staff training for the Consultation and Education program are those of the C&E director. Program staffing requires that attention be given to philosophical as well as practical considerations, especially when individuals from a traditional clinical role are to become consultants to the community. Both support and training should be provided to help clinician-consultants broaden their view of the helping relationship and deal with the many external, internal and personal factors that will impinge upon them in their new role.

An array of staffing and training issues will confront the C&E director, including such aspects as specialist versus generalist skills, clinical versus educational orientation, and professional credentials versus paraprofessional training. It would be dishonest to say that such issues will not, in part, be decided by the attitude, beliefs and desires of the C&E director. Yet, the needs of the community and the purposes of the C&E program must also receive serious attention. Ideally, a blend of clinician-consultants, educators, generalists, specialists and paraprofessionals would make for an exciting, multifaceted staffing pattern. In reality, this ideal is rarely possible to implement as financial constraints and, more important, service needs may not support a staffing pattern with these characteristics.

If one seeks to deliver quality consultation and education services, then one must build a quality staff. While this statement holds true for all center programs, it must be emphasized for C&E. Staff of the C&E program are the most visible of all CMHC staff due to the nature of their community roles. Indeed, the very image of the community mental health center can rise or fall based upon the behavior and perceived competence of C&E staff. The responsibilities accompanying a consultant or educator role are significant. Equally significant, however, are the opportunities for broad impact upon the mental health of the community.

Chapter 4

FINANCING CONSULTATION
AND EDUCATION

DAVID R. RITTER

THE topic of financing Consultation and Education frequently
provokes immediate discussion about sources of funding
and how those sources can be tapped. Certainly, the question of
"Where are the resources?" is a central question; but for the developing Consultation and Education program it is premature to
address this question first. The discussion and resolution of two
issues should take precedence to any efforts of actual acquisition
of funds: (1) the overall policy of the community mental health
center as it relates to the issue of free services versus fee for services; and (2) an examination of the values and attitudes of the
C&E director and staff regarding their role in securing funds for
the program.

INITIAL CONSIDERATIONS

An original concept of the community mental health center
movement of the early 1960s was the availability of services for
all individuals regardless of their ability to pay. Even today, centers continue that policy for their clinical services, as evidenced
by the existence of sliding fee scales that link reimbursement for
services to such variables as family income, family size and perhaps
even a consideration of outstanding debts on the part of the client.
A major rationale in support of the concept of sliding fee scales
is the substantial financial support for community mental health

centers provided through the grant structures of the National Institute of Mental Health. Thus, federal funding subsidizes the cost of services to clients. Where Consultation and Education is concerned, however, there is real question as to the legitimacy of a sliding fee scale approach. Through Public Law 94-63, the Community Mental Health Center's Ammendments, and its successor, Public Law 96-398, the Mental Health Systems Act, the legitimacy of Consultation and Education has been established as an integrated service of community mental health centers. Regrettably, federal dollars have not accompanied this federal sanctioning of C&E. Given this reality, the community mental health center needs to define its own policy on fees for C&E services. Generally, policies for established Consultation and Education programs do not reflect a sliding scale concept but instead seek reimbursement for services at a level commensurate with the actual cost of providing services. At the same time, flexibility for the delivery of free services to those C&E target populations which have been established as high priority but for whom it is clear that levels of reimbursement will be minimal can be maintained.

A second prerequisite to the exploration of actual income sources is an assessment of the attitudes and beliefs of the C&E staff themselves. To attain a financially solvent C&E program, staff must believe in the inherent value of the services that they deliver, with this value being reflected in dollars and cents.

Two of the most frequently voiced comments about Consultation and Education are that Consultation and Education programs cannot be financially self-supporting and that C&E programs have a very low priority when compared to other clinical programs of the center. Many individuals view these comments as mutually exclusive when, indeed, they are interrelated. Within many community mental health centers, C&E programs *do* have a low priority. This is not necessarily because the center director or the governing board are opposed to Consultation and Education as methods of service delivery but is due to the financial constraints of center resources, which pose a barrier to the development of C&E. Unfortunately, this financial barrier can all too readily become translated by staff into a statement to the effect of "if the center really believed in Consultation and Education, the money would be found to support it." This attitude approaches a belief that the center director has $50,000 or so stashed in a bottom desk drawer. In actuality, the problem is an attitudinal problem of remaining dependent instead of C&E asserting independence. A characteristic of this attitude is that C&E staff attend to programming while abdicating responsibility for the financing of C&E. Among all of the center's programs, clinical and C&E alike, there is probably no program that expects to deliver nonreimbursable services and projects a level of dependency as much as Consultation and Education. There is only one solution to this problem, that being that C&E programs *must* begin to assume responsibility for themselves, both fiscally as well as programmatically.

As serious consideration is given to the issue of priorities, it becomes quickly apparent that priorities are established as much upon fiscal solvency as upon philosophical orientation. Within an era of decreasing financial support, fiscal stability becomes a prime concern. Clinical services frequently have priority over C&E services *because* clinical services generate income. Compensation for services is an integral component of the therapeutic encounter. Similarly, service value should become as much a tenet for Consultation and Education as it is for clinical services, and it is critical that C&E staff begin to reflect this philosophy in their beliefs. Where C&E services begin to exist strictly on a fee-for-service basis or are provided through meaningful monetary contracts, C&E programs also begin to acquire a higher priority within the center. As C&E programs reach a point of generating substantial income for the center, their priority status may begin to reach parity with clinical programs. Certainly, C&E programs will require some level of subsidy by the center itself, but in reality, there are few programs within any center that are truly self-supporting. As efforts are made to increase the financial support of C&E services, and as the level of center subsidization of those services decreases, the assurance of the continued existence or even expansion of the Consultation and Education program is likewise increased. As has been repeatedly stressed in the chapter on organizational structure, it is the director of Consultation and Education who is the key to unlocking this problem, and it is for this reason that the authority and responsibility invested in this individual need to be substantial. The sources of monetary support for the C&E program are many, but before they can be meaningfully tapped, the basic values and beliefs of the C&E staff themselves must become oriented toward the assumption of personal responsibility for the financial support of their own positions and program.

CRITICAL CONCEPTS OF FUNDING

Within the arena of financial solvency, the Consultation and Education program must address a number of critical concepts. Initially, center policy and C&E program attitudes must be established around the issue of fee for service versus free service. Concurrently, where fee for service is required, the C&E staff must assume personal responsibility for being constantly aware of potential sources of monetary support, and they must actively explore such sources when they become available. The Consultation and Education program will have to spend money to make money. At one level this means that when the initial C&E development occurs under the auspices of federal grant support, a certain portion of grant-supported staff time should be devoted to efforts of securing funds to assure the delivery of C&E services beyond the period of grant support. Indeed, this is one of the major purposes of the seed money concept. Unfortunately, it is all too often relegated to a minor role, if it is attended to at all. Planning for continuation of funding beyond the period of grant support should be initiated almost immediately upon the receipt of any grant rather than waiting until the C&E program is in the final year of grant support to begin frantically to seek and develop alternative monetary sources. Some federal grant programs are quite explicit in their emphasis that one of the major goals of the grant supported program should be the development of continuation monies. For NIMH grant structures, however, this is seldom an emphasized point. Therefore, it becomes incumbant upon the C&E staff to establish continuation as a goal for themselves. At a second level, spending money to make money may mean that a capital investment needs to be made in the Consultation and Education program. More frequently than not, this takes the form of spending money to enable the program to develop a new direction by addressing needs of a target population that have not previously been an area of focus for the C&E program. For example, should one seek to develop consultation or management training for business and industry, there is a great deal more involved than simply approaching a business and offering services. Business and industry speak a management language rather than the jargon of human services, and they seek consultants and trainers who are familiar with both this language and the organizational structures, strengths and problems of the business world. C&E staff seeking to enter business and industry will require additional specialized training. Initial contacts need to be developed with the target business or industry, and meaningful relationships need to be established from which program presentations and financial negotiations can occur. If the C&E program is to have a management training emphasis, actual training modules themselves need to be developed, piloted and updated. All of these functions take time and cost money, and the monetary support of these development functions will fall to the C&E program. The potential for income to the C&E program, over time, is likely to be significant if serious attention is given to the development of the service. During the interim, however, the C&E program needs to make a capital investment in itself to realize potential income that would accrue from future contracts with business and industry. This capital investment approach is a method that is used on a daily basis by business and industry throughout the country. However, it will require attitudinal changes and adjustments on the part of the Community Mental Health Center, since CMHCs rarely view themselves from a business perspective.

The strength and vitality of the Consultation and Education program rest with its staff and their feelings of job security, support and financial reward, feelings that are directly linked to staff motivation and performance. Should a C&E program find itself with limited financial resources, either as part of its initial development or as a result of a centerwide financial crisis, the C&E program may want to consolidate its efforts. Programs confronted with financial restraints have two choices: to maintain the existing diversification of services and all existing staff, thereby operating the program on a shoestring; or to eliminate some services of the program and with them one or perhaps two staff positions. Admittedly, this is a very difficult choice. The most common occurrence is that a decision is made to operate the program on a shoestring either to protect the job security of staff or in the unrealistic hope that monies will be found to sustain the program. While such a decision is frequently made in support of staff needs for continued employment, the decision can be less than optimal, since operating on a shoestring is frequently accompanied by a curtailment of staff fringe benefits, training programs, monies to support attendance at professional conferences, etc. Curtailments may also be reflected in decreased staff raises or increases in staff work loads. While such curtailments may avoid the elimination of one or more positions within the C&E program, they may also seriously affect the motivation and performance of staff. Over time, this is a far more serious consequence than staff layoff. Consolidation, on the other hand, embodies the premise that the program is more important than any of its staff. The termination of one or more C&E services with its corresponding staff is deemed preferable than operating on a shoestring in responding to a financial crisis. Staff who continue to be part of the C&E program are not merely maintained but rather continue to receive all of the benefits and financial compensation that are appropriate.

The last critical funding concept concerns itself with the ability to identify potential sources of financial support. Knowing where sources of support exist and when those resources become available is sometimes more difficult than the actual application for or acquisition of funds. This is especially true with state or federal grants. Two useful methods for identifying funding sources and for becoming cognizant of grant authorized monetary levels and deadlines for grant applications include periodicals, notably the *Federal Register* and the *Commerce and Business Daily*. If one is serious in obtaining grant support for Consultation and Education, a subscription to one or both of these publications is well worth the annual subscription cost. These publications identify federal funding departments and also delineate amounts of money appropriated, the average monetary amount expected to be granted per application, the number of applications to be funded, deadlines for grant applications, where to obtain application packets and, most important, the intent or purpose for which grant funds are expected to be used. Another method for keeping abreast of newly developing grant sources is through personal contact with the staffs of state or district legislative leaders. Many community mental health centers have demonstrated the value of a trip to Washington for the purpose of establishing personal contact with legislative aides of their senators and representatives. Opportunity is provided for personal contact and for sharing information about the community mental health center, its programs, and the areas of interest for future service development. Subsequent to these personal visits, it is well to maintain periodic telephone contact with legislative aides both as a reminder of the center's interests and also to obtain an update on current or pending legislation that might be a source of grant support. On a state or local level, the development of ongoing contacts with key individuals of state Departments of Mental Health, Social and Rehabilitation Services, Corrections and Education may provide benefit both for information of funding sources and to keep abreast of new directions or philosophies within those departments. Maintaining ongoing contact with various state departments can also occur through the C&E Director or staff participating on state committees or advisory councils within their area of expertise. This range of functions constitutes an investment of capital in the C&E program, since advisory council or committee participation time will decrease time that would otherwise be devoted to delivery of local services. An investment of time and resources is necessary for the Consultation and Education program to assume a pro-active role in its own financial future.

RELATIONSHIP OF PROGRAM GOALS TO FINANCIAL RESOURCES

The Consultation and Education program's existing and future goals should serve as the guideline for the exploration of funds toward the program attaining its goals. An initial step in this planning process is for the C&E program to define its present goals based upon existing resources and staff expertise and also to define its future directions. It is helpful if these future goals are prioritized in some fashion, particularly if attainment of one goal is dependent upon the prior attainment of another goal. The development of definitions and goals is at the very heart of a planned rather than haphazard Consultation and Education program. However, future goals and directions retain their meaningfulness only when actual implementation closely follows the plan. "Chasing the buck" is not conducive to a well-planned C&E program, for it can lead to a piecemeal development of C&E services that may bear little relationship to one another. Therefore, when a funding source for a future program is identified, funds should only be actively pursued if the necessary prerequisite goals and services have already been established. A conscious choice *not* to pursue a funding source, based upon a well-developed C&E plan, is appropriate, but it may also be difficult. Yet, it is important to try not to "chase the buck" if one hopes to develop a pattern of services that reflects more than simply the pattern of available funding.

The planning, goal setting and prioritization for the future development of services within the Consultation and Education program bears relationship not only to funding through grant mechanisms but also to the diversification of funding mechanisms to be sought by the program. If a Consultation and Education program has established primary prevention as its focus, it will have little need to explore financial support areas such as third party funding. If, on the other hand, a C&E program has identified early identification and intervention for individuals experiencing mild emotional distress as one of its major objectives, then it would be natural for the C&E program to seek third party sources. Depending upon its purposes for existence, the C&E program may seek to develop one, two or many avenues of monetary support. The working rule should be planning first, funding second. In this manner, the C&E program can better define its interest to significant individuals and can focus its efforts more meaningfully on those sources of potential funding that relate directly to its areas of interest. Effective planning, goal setting, prioritization and charting of future service development are at the very heart of a planned approach toward the financial solvency of the Consultation and Education program.

SOURCES OF FINANCIAL SUPPORT

Methods for financing Consultation and Education can be as varied as the many types of C&E services themselves. For ease of discussion, however, they will be grouped into four categories: grants, contracts, consumer fees and sources of local support. Of the four categories, grants and contracts are perhaps the most stable funding mechanisms, since they have a designated monetary amount and the reliability factor of being at least year long. In the case of many grants, longevity is even greater. Consumer fees, on the other hand, are a variable funding source, fluctuating from month to month depending on the level of services delivered. Other sources of local support may or may not exist within a given community, and acquiring funds from this category usually depends upon whether the community mental health center is state affiliated or private nonprofit.

Grants

In past years, grants have been a major source of financial support of Consultation and Education programs. Indeed, the very existence of C&E services within many community mental health centers would not have otherwise occurred without federal grant support. Today, the free flow of federal grant monies is no longer available. The major community mental health center legislation of the 1980s, the Mental Health Systems Act, recognized the value of C&E services and established grant mechanisms for the support of programs aimed at the prevention of mental illness, the promotion of mental health, and other non-revenue-producing services. The Mental Health Systems Act also emphasized the importance of linkage with other community service providers toward a goal of developing an integrated community service system. However, "...for everything there is a season," and as seasons change, so too do administrations.

The presidential election of 1980 marked a major shift in the philosophy and involvement of the federal government in the support of human and social service programs. With the Federal Budget Reconciliation Act of 1981, all federal community mental health center legislation was repealed, and with this action, the potentials for monetary support of C&E services embodied in the Mental Health Systems Act ceased to exist.

Today, federal monies are allocated to the state under a system known as block grants. The state, in turn, becomes the funding authority with monies being distributed based upon state priorities. For the next few years, federal monies will continue to flow to community mental health centers that were grant recipients of NIMH funds at the time of this change to the block grant system. However, these monies are short lived. It becomes essential for C&E programs to view this continuing federal support as *transitional funding* and to begin to seek alternative sources of revenue.

Despite the major changes in the federal support role of human service programs, there are a few sources of grant support that continue to be in effect and available to C&E programs. NIMH has retained a small capacity to support applied research through its Division of Extramural Research and its Small Grants Program, which is specifically designed to support the piloting of small projects or to capitalize on unanticipated research opportunities. The U.S. Office of Education continues to maintain a commitment to the development of model/demonstration programs under its Office of Special Education, Rehabilitation Services Administration, and National Institute of Handicapped Research. Grants awarded by these federal agencies are more restrictive in nature inasmuch as they require a defined program evaluation component through which the effectiveness of model or demonstration programs can be documented. The majority of these grant structures emphasize innovative service approaches to individuals with handicapping conditions. Since such innovative delivery systems can include consultative, educational or early intervention methods, they continue to represent a source of financial support for C&E. Realistically, the number of annual grant awards are few, and the application process is intensively competitive. Resultantly, federal grants should no longer be considered as the core funding method for C&E but as only supplemental support.

Not to be overlooked within this area of grants are monies available from the state. With block grant funds going directly to the states, many states, in turn, have developed their own grant programs as a way of passing on monies to local service agencies. Mini-grants have flourished under this practice, and although the amount of dollars attached to any one mini-grant is limited, the application process is often far less complex and cumbersome than formerly existed under the federal system.

Contracts

Contracts with state or local agencies should be a substantial source of financial support for the Consultation and Education program. Contracts with state agencies frequently involve formula grant monies that are provided to states and, in turn, allocated to local service providers under the auspices of a contractual agreement. Drug abuse prevention and treatment through the National Institute of Drug Abuse, alcohol prevention and treatment through the National Institute of Alcoholism and Alcohol Abuse and the prevention of crime and delinquency through the Law Enforcement Assistance Adminstration are but a few examples of service areas supported by state contracts. State tax-based monies, appropriated to support state Departments of Mental Health or Hygiene, are sources of support for community mental health centers and, depending on the particular state plan for mental health services, may also have potential for use by Consultation and Education. State Departments of Education or Special Education are another source of support for C&E services that are provided to school systems.

The development of contracts with local social service agencies, schools, businesses and industries or other organizations is an area over which the Consultation and Education program can exercise control. C&E services should be provided under a contract that defines both the objectives and time frames for services as well as the monetary compensation for those services. Preferably, local contracts should be developed for a minimum of one year. Contract income will depend on the level of services to be provided. The development of local contracts depends as much upon the C&E program having a meaningful service to offer to the consultee organization as it does upon the art of negotiation itself.

There can be pitfalls inherent in the development of local contracts. Potentially, conflict can arise between consultee needs and

C&E program goals as, for example, a school system seeking to contract for consultation services for its teachers to help them manage behavior problems in the classroom, but the hidden agenda of the consultant is to seek to modify the organizational climate of the school. When a conflict is foreseen between a consultee's request and the C&E program's philosophy and goals, it is necessary to address those conflicts prior to the delivery of services. If resolution cannot be obtained, the C&E program faces the choice of modifying its own philosophy to provide the services requested by the consultee or to inform the consultee that the request cannot be met in a meaningful way by the C&E program and that, perhaps, a service provider other than the CMHC would be more appropriate. A second pitfall that exists in contract development is the offering of an initial free consultation service for the purposes of gaining systems entry. The willingness of a consultee organization to assume the costs of services is a direct reflection of the perceived value of the services and the priority and importance that the consultee places on those services. A consultee organization that is willing to accept services at no cost but at the same time would be unwilling to pay for services is providing a clear message that the services may be useful but that the consultee could certainly manage without them. Subtle implications of verbal statements of consultee organizations cannot be overlooked during contract negotiations so as to avoid a situation whereby free services provided initially are either continued at no cost during subsequent years or are not continued at all. This issue of monetary contracts for services should be addressed from the start with any consultee organization. While consultants and educators frequently cite one of the purposes of their role as "giving away their skills," this phrase cannot be taken too literally.

Consumer Fees

Consumer fees, as distinct from contractual monies, are generated through registration fees for community education workshops and courses or through self-pay or third party reimbursement for early intervention programs targeted at high risk populations. Each of these areas will be addressed separately.

Registration cost/fees for educational courses can generate income to help offset the cost of offering educational programs.

Admittedly, income derived from workshop/course registration fees is not large, primarily because of the limits placed on the number of individuals enrolling in a given workshop, and this income may not offset the total costs of providing a program. Yet, consumer fee income does meet some of those costs. Many C&E programs define a preestablished level of subsidy that is acceptable for community education courses, as for example, a decision that consumer fees must reach a level of reimbursing the salary costs of the workshop leader. The C&E program itself then subsidizes the cost of preparatory time, advertising, facilities, etc. Establishing a predetermined level of educational program subsidy allows the C&E program to better establish fee structures for educational programs and defines a criterion by which a decision can be made to offer the course or whether the course must be cancelled. This method seeks to avoid an inordinate drain of C&E resources on the part of educational courses and also establishes guidelines under which community educators can function with greater clarity. At the same time, community education programs retain their flexibility as, for example, the ability to offer an educational program even if consumer fees have not met the preestablished income level as long as consumer fees for other educational courses have comparably exceeded the prerequisite level. Flexibility allows educational courses to be targeted specifically at low income populations, since other community education offerings during the year are likely to generate a greater than expected amount of consumer fees that can, in turn, subsidize other programs.

The second area of consumer fees is that of self-pay or third party reimbursement for early intervention services. Before these services are tapped, however, the C&E program must realize that it is offering an early intervention rather than prevention service and that those services are under a medical model. Early intervention programs in reality do not greatly differ from group therapy programs, as participants in both early intervention and group therapy programs are in the midst of emotional distress. Intervention programs can be a legitimate role of the C&E program as long as C&E has defined early intervention as part of its purpose and function. The intervention itself would likely combine educational and therapeutic approaches, and legitimately, third party reimbursement can be sought to support the costs of early intervention as long as there is identified emotional distress on the part of participants. Additionally, the required physician supervision and record keeping associated with the medical model need to be provided. Third party reimbursement would not become a component of a community education program that is simply designed to educate the community at large rather than address the specific emotional needs of individuals actually experiencing emotional distress. Some of the more common early intervention target populations include parents of Sudden Infant Death children, children of divorced parents, or children of mentally ill parents.

Early intervention programs within C&E cannot be discussed without attention being given to the potential conflict that might arise between the C&E program and clinical services. As a C&E program enters the area of early intervention, it also runs the risk of encroaching upon the territory of clinical services. To avoid conflict, the C&E program and the clinical programs need to define who, will do what, for whom. Clarification should involve a discussion of early intervention programs that will be provided by clinical services and early intervention programs that will be under the auspices of C&E.

Other Local Support

Other sources of support include income from foundations, revenue sharing, United Way, fund-raising events and monies that may accrue to the center through county or local taxes. The overall center, rather than any specific program, is usually the recipient of monies from these sources, and funds are frequently used to offset administrative and support costs to the center. Of the many funding sources within this category, county or local tax dollars would have the greatest significance and, should these funds be available to the center, it would be important for the Director of C&E to advocate for a reasonable and proportionate share of unallocated monies for the C&E program.

Seeking financial support from foundations can frequently be an arduous and disappointing experience. Community mental health centers seldom seek to develop programs that will either have national significance or function as the cutting edge in pioneering a new development. However, these are the types of programs that foundations seek to support. For the average community mental health center, foundations are not a viable source of funding. Should a center wish to seek foundation support, it is necessary to be cognizant of the great deal of time and effort that will be needed in this venture, not the least of which is involved in proposal writing and travel to the foundation locale for the purposes of conferring with the foundation's executive administrator.

Fund-raising events have become fashionable in recent years, and it is unusual that a week goes by without some association or cause undertaking an event. For community mental health centers, fund-raising events are likely to have the greatest success when they are linked to a one-time event, such as the building or renovation of the center's facilities. Fund raising is not a solid source of support for ongoing programming. Realistically, the financial needs of the community mental health center would seem to be better served through center participation as a United Way agency, since this communitywide fund-raising event has the specific purpose of supporting social services within the community and offers the availability of continued support over a number of years.

THE STATE OF FINANCIAL AFFAIRS

In attempting to develop Consultation and Education programs, and in doing so project toward the future, it is also useful to retrospectively view C&E to discern trends in staffing and financing. Annually, the National Institute of Mental Health surveys all federally funded community mental health centers to assess the status and well-being of the system. Evolving from a series of NIMH Annual Reviews from the mid- to late 1970s has been a compilation of the National Data and Trends for C&E Services (Hassler, 1978).

From a historical perspective, efforts devoted to Consultation and Education have been progressively declining. In the early 1970s, 4.8 percent of all CMHC staff hours were devoted to C&E. Only 3.2 percent of staff hours were delivered by C&E by the end of the decade. This represents a decrease of fully one-third of C&E

service hours. Nationally, the staffing pattern of Consultation and Education programs has also fluctuated. C&E programs averaged 3.4 full-time equivalent staff during the early 1970s and declined to a low of 3.0 full-time equivalent staff in the late 1970s. The C&E staffing pattern trend somewhat reflects the federal government's commitment to Consultation and Education. In 1975, Public Law 94-63 specifically identified a need for the development of Consultation and Education services and marked the beginning of the C&E grant mechanism. Community mental health centers responded to this initiative by increasing their C&E staffing patterns. During subsequent years, however, verbal support for C&E far outweighed financial support. With the 1980 passage of the Mental Health Systems Act there was an indication of renewed recognition and support for Consultation and Education, although recognition again exceeded monetary support.

Reliance upon federal funding for the development and sustenance of Consultation and Education is apparent in the National Data and Trends Survey. During the early 1970s, the average monetary receipts (other than grants) for Consultation and Education services across all federally funded centers totaled a mere $3100. By the late 1970s, average receipts for C&E services totaled $11,000, a rather insignificant increase in the development of alternative funding sources given the inflationary times of the mid-1970s. Considering receipts from other than grant funds from the perspective of the number of years of C&E program operation, it is evident that Consultation and Education has not assumed a sufficient level of responsibility for its own financial solvency. By the late 1970s, the average receipts across all C&E programs averaged $11,000: C&E programs in their first or second year averaged $6,000; programs in their third or fourth years averaged $6,000; programs in their sixth and seventh years averaged $11,000 and programs in their eighth and ninth years averaged $21,000. The National Trends Data indicate that Consultation and Education programs do not begin to increase their levels of local support until their sixth or seventh years of operation. Concerted and probably frantic efforts to obtain local support occur during the eighth or ninth years of operation, a period by which federal staffing grant support is terminated. It appears that Consultation and

Education programs feel little pressure or incentive to develop alternative sources of funding during their initial years of operation, perhaps as a result of the feeling of security that grants can provide. Only when C&E programs begin to feel the squeeze of declining grant support do they actively begin to seek alternative resources. Indeed, the data suggest that programs are successful in this endeavor, since the average C&E program better than triples its nongrant funding base when it finally feels a need to do so. It is regrettable that such efforts are not made earlier and that monies that are available within the community are not more fully used.

It is not surprising that many Consultation and Education programs are perceived as low priority. Indeed, *any* program whose income levels comprised such a small percentage of total center receipts would be perceived as such. It is interesting to note that nationally the combined income of the ten greatest income producing C&E programs still comprised only 10.5 percent of all income of those ten centers. Even at its best, income derived from Consultation and Education services is but a small percentage of the total income of any community mental health center. Nevertheless, the levels of income of these top ten C&E programs are such that they offer greater self-sufficiency and solvency than the majority of C&E programs, which assume little responsibility for their own financing.

THE ART OF FINANCIAL SOLVENCY

The solicitation of monies to support Consultation and Education programs is more an art than a science. There are times when requests or applications for financial aid are awarded as much upon the basis of personal contact, center image, and letters of support as upon the quality of the application itself. This is not to say that the format of the request itself is not important. Indeed, the clear and concise writing of any financial application is crucial. Many well-intentioned and carefully designed programs are rejected by potential funding sources. Sometimes this is a result of severe competition for limited funds, but it can also be failure of the financial application itself. Important sections of financial applications sometimes receive only perfunctory attention. These include the quality and range of letters of support for the grant application and efforts to make the personal contact that can sometimes have a positive impact upon the receptiveness of the application.

Grantsmanship is an art, and there are many books on the market today that seek to teach this art. For the uninitiated individual with limited knowledge of grants, books can be useful to provide a broad overview of the grant process. Beyond that initial perspective, however, the value of text is limited. Workshops or seminars on grant writing provide a greater level of information and expertise and also have the value of participants being able to ask very specific questions that directly relate to specific needs for information. Perhaps the best but most under used method of gaining information on grant writing is actually to obtain copies of grant applications that have been submitted and funded. This can be more difficult than it sounds, since grant applications are often well guarded and protected. A useful first step would be to seek out all of the prior grant applications that have been developed by one's own center and carefully review those applications for their structure and format. Considering the literary and writing skills of various center staff to determine which individuals write concisely and poignantly and to solicit their participation in the actual writing of grant applications can be most helpful. It is also useful to contact the agency to which the grant application will be submitted and to request technical assistance on the application process itself. This procedure is a clear indication of intent to work closely with the funding source toward meeting the goals and objectives of the grant application, should it receive favorable response and approval.

In the same manner that one would diversify one's own investments, so too should diversification be sought in the financing of the Consultation and Education program. Income sources should be blended among grants, contracts, fees and other resources. The degree to which diversification of funding occurs will be dependent upon the diversification of the C&E services themselves, as planning and program development are directly linked with funding. Should grants provide a substantial portion of the C&E funding base, careful attention must be given to the life of those grants in order that two or more major grants do not terminate within the same year. Grants of limited duration, such as one-year grants, should be used only as start-up monies or should not be sought at all. C&E program dependency on "soft" monies is a sure way of courting programmatic and fiscal disaster. Although the budget may balance within a given fiscal year, the illusion of financial solvency is created when, in fact, fiscal stability does not exist. Planning for the continuation of finances beyond the period of grant support should begin with the first year of any grant. Last, the concept of capital investment, spending money to make money, should become a planned approach to the development of C&E services that have a future potential for financial security.

The future economic realities surrounding community mental health dictate that financial management of the Consultation and Education program be on a par with the management of services and staff. To do less merely courts disaster, as with the loss of monies also comes the demise of that array of services that truely represents the original intent and purpose of community mental health.

REFERENCES

Hassler, F. *Current national data and trends for C&E services.* The National Institute of Mental Health: The Staff College, November 1978.

Chapter 5

THE PROCESS OF CONSULTATION

JAMES B. DUFFEY, ELIZABETH GIRSHICK and
FRANCIS J. ROBINSON

*D*R. *Weaver grimaced as he put down the phone. Mr. Ferguson, the principal at the local high school, while attempting to be polite, had made it clear that he was disappointed with the quality of professional consultation services he was receiving from the center.*

As the Director of Consultation and Education Services of the mental health center, Dr. Weaver had been working steadily for five years to improve the quality of services. He had made major administrative changes, and the leadership of the various professional groups was now of excellent quality. There had also been staff changes among the social workers, psychologists, speech clinicians and others, and Dr. Weaver had been careful to select staff members with outstanding professional skills. He had instituted an efficient referral system, a strong in-service program and excellent clinical supervision and support for his staff. Still, one of the center's major clients continued to be dissatisfied.

On the phone, Mr. Ferguson complained about the services recently received from one of the center's psychologists. He had requested consultation with a group of his teachers to assist them in improving their classroom management techniques. Mr. Ferguson indicated that the teachers had reported that the psychologist appeared to be interested in helping with the problem but that there had been little awareness among the teachers concerning the psychologist's expertise to meet their needs. In fact, Mr. Ferguson was totally unaware of the psychologist's background until Dr. Weaver had described his qualifications and excellent skills on the phone. Mr. Ferguson reported that he was not confident that the psychologist really understood the request for help, since he provided services the teachers had not expected. In addition, the teachers were not sure whether or not the psychologist had completed his work or whether he would be returning to the school again. According to Mr. Ferguson, the teachers had simply done what they were told to do by the psychologist and had no involvement in planning intervention procedures with the psychologist. The teachers indicated that they had little faith in the psychologist's suggestions and, just as they had suspected, his suggestions had made very little difference. Just prior to Mr. Ferguson's call, the teachers had again asked the principal to find someone to help them with classroom management techniques.

A week earlier, the psychologist in question had reported to Dr. Weaver that he had successfully dealt with the consultation request and made specific recommendations to the teachers. When asked to provide direct services to children and parents, this same psychologist had been highly complimented. Of even more concern to Dr. Weaver was that he had heard similar complaints regarding other staff members in other professional disciplines. Yet, he had the same degree of confidence in their clinical skills as he did in the psychologist about whom Mr. Ferguson had complained.

Dr. Weaver was now deep in thought. Perhaps he had not adequately attended to the needs of his staff after all. While the clinical skills of his staff were excellent, they apparently had a need to learn more about the process of interacting with clients effectively and in ways that would provide client satisfaction. Perhaps, they needed training in the consultation process.

In reality, it would be rare today to find a service center with professional staff members as unaware of the consultation process as the psychologist was in the narrative above. More often we find that professionals have some knowledge of the consultation process, at least enough to keep from being grossly misunderstood in their work. Unfortunately, many lack formal training and supervision in the development of consultation skills. Also common is the professional with adequate knowledge of consultation who mysteriously does not take the time or provide the effort necessary to deliver high quality consultation services.

This chapter will focus on the consultation process involving mental health professionals who serve educational agencies and other similar groups. It should be noted that most of what is written here could just as well apply to other professional groups who are responsible for delivery of consultation services.

The chapter will deal with three major aspects of the consultation process. The first relates to gaining credibility for systems entry. How should the consultant present himself* to his clients? How can the consultant gain the confidence of the organization's administration and the direct consultee group? What should the consultant do to start the process correctly?

The second section of this chapter will examine the assessment of client needs. Typically, those requesting consultation will express a need or several needs. Sometimes they will be totally accurate, but on other occasions they will misidentify the needs or expect the consultant to assist in identifying needs.

A third section of this chapter will discuss the development and negotiation of consulting contracts, the need for such contracts in terms of establishing expectation, as tools for later evaluating the quality of the services rendered. Section III will also serve to point out the various issues and items that should be specified in a contract.

Finally, other issues crucial to the delivery of services under a consultation model will be presented. Some of the major issues include ethical considerations and personal concerns.

It is important to note that the discussion of the consultation process in this chapter is less than exhaustive. The issues selected for presentation were chosen because of their meaningfulness to the authors, who have all spent years delivering services through a consultation model from a mental health/education perspective.

---

*The use of the pronoun "he" throughout this chapter is for the purpose of simplification of writing and refers to "he" or "she" as may be applicable.

GAINING CREDIBILITY FOR SYSTEMS ENTRY

To gain credibility, the consultant's task is threefold. He must convince his consultees of the value of his assistance, the acceptability of his personal style and the consultee's need for his services. If he is successful in this preliminary effort, the tasks to follow will be completed more easily.

Expertise and Power

The potential consultee has probably been struggling with his problem for some time. Other intervention strategies, and possibly other consultants, have been tried. Because past efforts have not brought about the desired change, the consultee seeks a consultant who is perceived as having expertise relevant to the present problem. It would certainly be an unfortunate situation if a non-expert consultant accepted a role for which he was not qualified. This could possibly reinforce the consultees' waivering lack of faith in the consultation process and make them lose their motivation for continued efforts, in the belief that a solution to their problems is unlikely.

Failure to follow a procedure to establish credibility and expertise may result in heightened doubts about the probability of success on the part of consultees throughout the process; questioning of the consultant's approaches and actions; and uncertainty about the consultant's helpfulness, even in successful interventions. For example, despite Dr. Weaver's expert staff, his psychologist lacked credibility in the school setting, and this contributed to his lack of success.

The suggestion to establish credibility assumes that the consultant does have sufficient expertise in the problem area under question. Under no condition should the consultant misrepresent the expertise that he can bring to a given situation. He must be willing to admit when he is really not the best person for the job.

At the time of initial contact, the assignment must be viewed as a potential one for the consultant, since it may be determined that the relationship should not proceed. Lack of expertise on the part of the consultant or inability to establish an effective working relationship is a possible reason for termination. The consultant may then wish to assist the consultee in finding the proper expert. In other cases, it may be initially apparent to the consultant that a significant problem does not exist or that the existing problem is not solvable through consultation. Obviously, the latter conclusion should only be determined by a consultant with sufficient expertise to make that decision.

The initial "selling" of the consultant is an important step in determining subsequent interactions between the consultant and his clients. It is essential to set groundwork for a relationship that will establish the consultant not just as an authority figure but also as a valuable source of information and guidance. The consultant's value to a consultee increases when he is able to "sell" himself as an expert. Understanding the sources of one's power can aid in using it most effectively. The characteristics associated with expertise in the minds of various populations of consultees differ with the nature of the setting and the job to be done. French and Raven (1959) describe one kind of power, expert power, based on externals (such as affiliations, age, etc.) that help a consultant to create the image of being an expert. For example, an individual who is highly paid for his services may be thought of as a competent consultant by some before they become aware of his skills. Referent power, on the other hand, refers to the feeling of confidence in a consultant that may be evoked by virtue of similar attitudes and behaviors of his clients. While a consultant's credentials are almost always investigated during the hiring process, the sources of referent power often remain unknown until after the work has begun. In attempts to increase the strength of one's referent power, some consultants become involved in issues and activities with their consultees, either social or professional, unrelated to the project. Martin (1978), while stressing the importance of maximizing the consultant's aura of competence, questions the advisability of this tactic because of the possible effect of increasing referent power at the expense of losing expert status. Familiarity, Martin explains, lessens one's position of expert influence. Schowengerdt (Fine *et al.*, 1979) believes that the role of consultant's interpersonal skill is the main factor in determining the success of the process. Hander (Meyers *et al.*, 1977) further refined the definition of this needed interpersonal skill as the ability to foster mutual respect. Martin (1978) adds that the consultant's view of his consultees is also an important element in determining the climate for consultation. Thus, if the consultant does not have confidence in the abilities of his consultees, or views them as helpless or incompetent, he might consider rejecting the assignment.

As part of the introductory procedure, the consultant should describe his areas of expertise to increase the confidence others will have in his ability to provide the requested services. It is important that the consultant not assume that his expertise is known or be embarrassed to present his skills adequately. Failure to do so may result in the ultimate failure of the consultation relationship. The professional resume provided to the consultees and the initial interview with prospective consultees should review the consultant's educational and experiential background and indicate his theoretical and methodological orientation. It is helpful to offer to clients reports of previous successful similar assignments from which they may become aware of effective ways to use the consultant's services (Lombana, 1979). While the consultant is attempting to convince his customers of his talents and areas of expertise, it is also important for him to state any limitations of his own knowledge or circumstances that he feels may interfere with his optimally meeting the expectations of his consultees. Because of an individual's desire to present himself in the best light possible, professional limitations are rarely reported to potential clients.

Dealing With Power

In most consultation arrangements, the consultant is given some type of power. Those who give administrative power to an outside consultant will have to communicate this to the consultees to make it effective power. On the other hand, a consultant, in a collegial relationship with his clients, with no real authority over them, should only attempt to *recommend* or *suggest* problem modifications and technical changes. He must not assume a superior role if there is no actual power to support it, for that would alienate his consultees and might result in poor motivation and cooperation. Typically, the greater the degree of authority a consultant assumes in his role, the more accountable he will be concerning the outcome of the program implemented. If the project fails, blame will be placed on the consultant in a superior position, while co-workers are more likely to share responsibility with an advisory consultant. The role of the consultant and his line staff or ancillary position with an organization will vary according to the type of system and its administrative structure, its scope of influence and funding sources and, finally, according to the type of consulting problem encountered.

To promote cooperation, the consultant must clearly define his role in meeting prescribed goals. The goals should also be operationally defined in a consultation contract (to be discussed later) prior to the onset of the program. Within the field of mental health or education, the roles of the consultant will vary depending on whether the setting is a mental health center, hospital, school or private agency. The types of individuals *asking* for the services of a consultant and those *receiving* those services will also differ greatly. The authority of the persons requesting the consultation over those participating in the program will be a factor that also varies with each situation. The affiliation of the consultant will, in part, determine the tone of the working relationship. That he is employed by the same facility to which he is consulting, by an organization in an associated field, by an industry typically unrelated to mental health or education or is in private practice will greatly affect his power, authority and loyalties to the particular system being considered for consultation. The effects of his professional affiliation will relate to the consultees' attitude toward and previous experience with similar groups of professionals.

For a moment, let's consider the psychologist in our earlier example. As a staff member of the mental health center, he was an outsider to the school system. The role he played, while acceptable in other situations, did not meet the needs of this group of teachers. In this instance, knowledge of the consultation process may have made the results different.

Getting Consultees Involved

To create a climate of cooperation and avoid an image of superiority, the consultant should not suggest that consultees will receive services or merely participate in them. Such a presentation of services may elicit a passive involvement on the part of the consultees (Lombana, 1979). In fact, it is important to get consultees truly involved and invested in the consultation project.

A consultant must discover his consultees' motivation for participation in the program with him. Is it something that *they* requested of the administration or is it mandated by the administration? If they are forced to participate, they may suspect that it is an evaluation designed to reveal shortcomings in their work. Suggestions will be responded to as criticisms. The consultant will have to deal with resistance. The nature of resistance can relate to the amount of power the consultant is given. Thus, a consultant who has firm administrative authority over his consultees may experience passive resistance, while a less powerful consultant may be faced with more active negativism.

Obviously, it is ideal to be invited into a situation where services have been requested by the consultees, and typically, objectives are much easier to accomplish under these conditions. However, this is often not the case. In these situations, it is advisable not to plunge into the actual project without first dealing with the feelings of the consultee group. If resistance or hostility is encountered, the consultant may wish to seek solutions and recommend them to the administration or the consultees. If possible solutions are not apparent, the consultant may simply accept the concerns of the consultee group but proceed with the project while communicating the understanding that despite negative feelings, there is still much that can be gained through the project, either individually, by the consultee group, organizationally or in all of these areas.

An approach that consistently seems to reduce resistance is to encourage consultee input in planning, revising and criticizing at the beginning of the project. One way that resistance is frequently expressed by consultees is through interruption or inattention at meetings with the consultant. An effective way to combat this behavior is to redirect their energy by giving them active developmental work to do instead of just allowing them to listen and to elicit and respond to their questions and skeptical comments.

One type of resistance to be anticipated is resistance to change (Hartley, 1979) in both theory and practice. Lombana (1979) found that consultees can react with resistance to unfamiliar systematic approaches. An attempt to change an ongoing system may be interpreted as a reflection of inadequacy on those who designed it and work within it. Introduction of new techniques and the assimilation of new ideas require education, practice and effort greater than that necessary to remain in familiar, comfortable work patterns. The consultant *must* justify the need for his recommended changes and allow consultees to determine their own good reasons for implementing them.

McGregor (1960) points out that individuals usually possess the motivation and desire to do good work. Therefore, if they perceive the need for their involvement, consultees can frequently be expected to follow through with dedication. The consultant must never neglect the needs and opinions of the consultee in favor of concentrating on his own notion of the problem and its solution (Abidin, 1977), for it is consultees' output that ultimately determines the success or failure of the contract goals.

It has been suggested that the consultant-consultee relationship is a crucial factor in determining the results of consulting projects (Lombana, 1979). If relationships remain consistently negative, then the result of the project will most often be negative. The consultant who invests less than a strong effort in dealing with relationship problems is not a good consultant, simply because he is not an optimally effective one.

One method for sharing relevant information, defining the role of the consultant and gathering data from which to organize the consultation program is the inclusion of training sessions into the initial planning stages. The consultant can use this forum to present his ideas to the consultee group and to explain why he typically recommends specific procedures or changes and how he will go about achieving goals. If the consultees understand the rationale for the technique applied in the intended program, they will better be able to work toward desired objectives and will be more cooperative in so doing.

Consultees are a source of information to the consultant in terms of describing the needs of the setting, identifying the providers of service, identifying client groups and revealing what factors will limit the introductions of certain modifications. Thus, they can provide an understanding of the ongoing realities of the situation to the consultant, who most often is entering the system fleetingly, to complement his store of generalized impressions and allow for the implementation of an optimal program. Because the consultees will emanate the changes, they must be involved in determining what changes will occur so as to maximize the probability that changes will be internalized and acted upon (Martin, 1978). The need for ongoing dialogue with the consultee group should not be underestimated. There are motivational gains to be achieved by "letting in" the consultees at the planning stages. By asking for consultee input, the consultant is publicly recognizing them as knowledgeable professionals with valid and valued opinions. By having them participate in planning the process of change, the consultant is allowing their perceptions of their needs to be expressed and included, fostering more personal investment in the changes to be made. Chandler (1980) advocates assuming roles of coprofessionals from the organizational phases of the consultation to the preparation of the plan of action. This assumes respect for the consultees' own skills and judgments. He also advises a consultant to maintain frequent contact with consultees to provide continued emotional support and technical guidance and to receive feedback as the recommendations actually begin to be implemented.

If system changes are seen only as the consultant's changes, then why should the consultees cooperate or implement these changes? Aren't they, in fact, seeing their old system discredited? When consultees see changes as something they have helped to foster, they can take ownership of those changes. They can perceive themselves as improving their old system and can support these changes without losing face. Obviously, a self-improvement plan will have a much higher probability of success with an existing staff than a plan that discredits an old system and brings in a new one. The successful consultant leaves his consultees with the feeling that they have improved things for themselves and that the consultant merely helped a little.

NEEDS ASSESSMENT

Before a formal needs assessment process begins, there has usually been discussion within the organization concerning needs from a technical, personal or other perspective. A consultant then is selected by the organization because there is a belief that he can help in remediating a preidentified set of needs. Typically, the consultant has already expended effort in gaining credibility and entering the system in relation to that set of needs. It may, in fact, turn out that the organization requesting services has correctly identified all of their needs, but often this is not the case. Thus, a formal needs assessment process should be pursued.

Another possibility can occur. Sometimes an organization desiring consultation assistance sees the primary work to be needs assessment. In this case, the contract for services will be negotiated before the formal needs assessment begins. Regardless of which activity takes precedence, the following tenets and concerns regarding needs assessment usually are applicable and should be pursued as carefully as possible.

In this chapter we have elected to discuss needs assessment prior to contract negotiation. Obviously, it is desirable that all needs be properly identified prior to the negotiation of the contract, but it is rare that the needs initially identified turn out to be all the needs that are eventually identified or that all the identified needs are properly and completely described. Even though it is suggested here that a formal needs assessment process be undertaken, it is with the understanding that needs assessment is a continuous process. Some needs assessment preceeds the formal needs assessment process by later updating the identified needs.

As noted, the organization requesting consultation may not have adequately described its needs. Originally described needs may be found to be symptomatic of another less visible disorder. A thorough needs assessment helps assure that the energy of the consultation effort is focused in a direction that will yield positive results.

When the consultant realizes that attention to an overt problem alone is superficial, he faces a dilemma. While easier to address, and possibly less threatening to the organization's structure, real and effective change will not result from concentration on only this particular facet of the situation. The consultant must reveal these findings to the organization that has sought consultation assistance. If he has employed a needs assessment technique that incorporates the suggestions of his consultees and has acknowledged the strengths of their present system of operation, mention of undisclosed weaknesses may not be as threatening to the consultees or as damaging to the course of the consultation. When a consultant delves deeper into the problem than initially anticipated, he must be willing either to take on the responsibility of a more in-depth project or to direct those who contracted for services to more appropriate resources. This suggests still another phase of the needs assessment function, the investigation of other support services or agencies that might be available to the consultee. Should the job prove bigger than anticipated, available funding and disciplinary responsibilities need to be considered to be able to recommend optimal intervention.

We have indicated that needs may turn out to be different than originally expected. One way for needs to be different is when the appropriate consultee turns out to be other than originally identified. For example, a school principal may request the services of a consultant with the identified need of speeding up the multidisciplinary team process of the school. The principal might feel that the expertise of team members is insufficient because the process is slow and few cases are fully addressed. The consultant, after studying the problem, might find that the multidisciplinary team process is slowed by policies and regulations promulgated by the principal himself. The consultee has thus changed. The consultant must redefine the need to the principal, and it is he who must behaviorally change if the multidisciplinary team process is to accomplish more in a shorter time. Obviously, these situations require special sensitivity and delicacy on the part of the consultant in seeking resolutions.

The Needs Assessment Process

Rather than going into excruciating detail on how a needs assessment process should be conducted, we will talk more about general issues concerning consultation.

Before the consultant is able to provide input, he should learn as much about the presenting problem as possible. Offering suggestions before such knowledge is acquired demonstrates a lack of respect for the consultee who has been seeking solutions for some time. Depending on the circumstances, it may be advisable to review written records, conduct surveys, interview individuals or groups and observe the work environment. Observing consultees in action in their own social and organizational systems can be a useful way of gaining understanding of the consultees' point of view and method of functioning (Cohen, 1964).

Since the consultees' request for consultation services is based on their perceptions of their needs, the consultant will find it useful to explore the history of the presenting problem and methods used in the past to deal with the issue. He will want to know what internal measures have been taken and what other resources have been tapped. He must research the outcome of each past strategy so as to prevent unproductive duplication of efforts. It would also be beneficial to attempt to analyze the personal factors contributing to the problem (lack of administrative support, personality factors, etc.) and try to capitalize on strengths and avoid similar pitfalls in the present effort.

A consultant must discover his consultees' motivation for participation. This is essential to estimate adequately the amount of responsibility they can be counted on to assume and their commitment to valid execution of the tasks required in the project. The issue will be discussed in greater depth later in this chapter. However, motivation of the consultee *is* a critical issue that should be initially explored at the time of needs assessment. Obviously, client motivations will change and must be continuously reassessed and attended to.

During the needs assessment phase, a recommended approach to the assessment of consultee motivation is the development and administration of a simple questionnaire. This approach has the advantage of providing the consultant with a global, if not detailed, perception of client motivation. If properly executed, it tends to be nonthreatening to the consultee group and can serve as a vehicle for initiating communication.

The consultant must become aware of the administrative structure of the school, hospital, industry or public agency for whom he is working, since it may be very different in each of these settings. Power will be officially designated by the administrative hierarchy and function according to an organizational plan. Some, however, will be dictated by purely political and negotiational motivations and, therefore, more difficult to reveal and deal with.

A consultant can study organizational charts and descriptions of departmental hierarchical structure, but some lines of power will never be known by a consultant because of short-term, fragmented observations.

Lombana (1979) warns that consultation cannot work well without administrative support. Administrators must be informed of the consultant's purposes and plans if their involvement and support are to be obtained. Administrators' needs and preferences must be considered and respected for the consultant to expect eventual implementation of his proposal.

A consultant must be careful to learn the legal guidelines governing the agency for which he is working. This is a necessary part of the needs assessment process. These include federal and state laws and regulatory conditions of funding or governmental sanction. The task includes not only discussing these with designated personnel but also a personal review of relevant documents. Through this procedure, the consultant can be sure changes proposed in consultation will comply with the legal regulations. The procedure will also aid in tactfully revealing and remediating any previous compromises of the intentions of the law. Such issues as the confidentiality and rights to services to which the agency's clients are entitled must be considered to avoid initiating changes or making recommendations that are in violation of the law or client's rights. If the project is focused on clients of a particular professional group, i.e. psychologists, physicians, police officers, their code of professional ethics should be reviewed.

When needs have been explored to the extent that the consultant is confident that at least the majority of needs have been identified, he is ready to begin thinking about intervention.

CONTRACT DEVELOPMENT AND NEGOTIATIONS

After it has been determined that consultation is appropriate, that a working relationship exists and that needs have been appropriately identified, an initial contract is negotiated. This contract provides the consultant with administrative sanction and support and outlines procedures and roles. Caplan (1970) writes that sanction must also be obtained from people in intermediate layers of the authority heirarchy and from the line workers of the institution as the consultant develops his successive roles. By seeking input from all concerned parties and involving them in the development of the plan, various individuals and groups know about the plan and have a personal commitment to support it.

Many consultation efforts have been judged as less than successful simply because an appropriate contract was not initially negotiated. The consultant must know exactly what he will be expected to do, and there should be sufficient communication between the consultant and consultee so that the procedures that will be followed in accomplishing objectives are familiar. The administration must know exactly what it will receive as a result of the consultation effort. False, unclear or unrealistic expectations are to be avoided. Such expectations may lead the consultee to perceive a successful effort as a failure.

The contract need not be highly technical or formal to be effective. In fact, such a contract may interfere with the consultation process by limiting flexibility. A working agreement, preferably in writing, is needed. This should contain general guidelines about the initial activities of fact-finding and discussion concerning the problem and the ability of the consultant and consultee to work together toward solving the problem. As the parties continue to work together, the contract may need to be amended. Different or additional needs or problems may be identified at some point, and the parties may wish to reassign priorities or place multiple problems in a hierarchy. Role functions and responsibilities may also change during the course of the consultation. For example, a teacher may contact a psychologist expressing a need for testing of a particular student because he presents behavioral difficulties in the classroom. While the psychologist in the opening narrative may believe that consultation with the teacher is all that is needed, it may be advisable to meet the teacher's expressed need so as to gain acceptance and establish rapport. Once established, the role of the consultant can develop and change.

Establishing Roles Within the Contract Framework

It is recommended that the notion of equal professionals with different perspectives working together to solve a problem be evident in the contract. The consultee ought to be free to either accept or reject the consultant's input, or the entire consultation agreement, with the consultant having no administrative authority for the consultee's behavior. Clarifying this issue can help greatly in reducing the consultee's anxiety and resistance as well as improving chances that the consultee will invest more of himself into the process. Obviously, this must be done in a nonthreatening way, and the consultant should reiterate his support for the consultee in his efforts.

The desired role one is expected to fill as a consultant in a particular consultative setting must be clear and ought to be included as part of a contract. This refers not only to the method of consultation to be used but also to the system of authority relationships and how the consultant must relate to it. To whom does the consultant report? It must be clear to the consultant if these individuals are to be superiors *for whom* he works; or is he in an advisory position to them as colleagues? The relationship of the consultant to his consultees, if they are not the same individuals who hired him, must also be determined. If he is given actual authority over the work of his consultees, the flavor of their interactions, and possibly their personal investments in the project will be different than if they are to function as co-workers. Giving authority to a consultant may provide for faster systematic change in a given situation. In others, it may actually be counterproductive because of staff resentment. In either case, less than desirable results may ensue from giving a consultant authority over existing staff. What happens when the consultant leaves? If change has been accomplished by direction, these changes may quickly crumble in the consultant's absence.

An individual who is functioning as a consultant to others within his own organization must be particularly clear in defining his role, especially if it conflicts with the usual way he interacts with and works with other employees. Fine et. al. (1979) indicated that the "spell" of the consultation contract might provide an advantage to the consultant brought in from outside of an organization, not only because of his perceived expert power but also because he enters the system unencumbered by previous hierarchical status. Obviously, the "inside" consultant may find himself at a considerable disadvantage in his own organization. If lines of authority and/or communication are variations of the way they usually are within the organization and are not properly defined, the inside consultant may be ignored and resented. Despite his expertise or the value of his advice, he faces adversity. Conversely, factors such as the knowledge of the power structure (both formal and informal) can be an asset to an "inside" consultant.

Organizational Commitment

As soon as possible and practical, the consultant should obtain details of the organization's commitments with regard to time, space, personnel and budget. The consultant needs to know what limitations exist and what channels of communication are available. This information should be included in the contract at the initial planning stages. The absence of expected resources is one sure way to defeat an otherwise well planned consulting effort.

Financial Aspects of the Contract

The financial arrangements must be clearly stated in the consultation agreement. In some cases there are overriding agreements between agencies that one will provide services to the other without a specific fee for particular services. While financial arrangements might not be described in such a consulting contract, it is wise to include some description of the quantity and depth of services to be provided out of existing resources.

In a fee-for-service arrangement, there are a number of possibilities for payment that might be considered. The consultant might be hired on an hourly or daily basis or might be reimbursed for work completed or objectives achieved. A retainer or retainer-plus (retainer plus provision for additional reimbursement should additional services become necessary) might be negotiated. In all cases, amounts and dates of payment should be clearly negotiated and stated in the consultation contract.

Confidentiality of Information

Issues relating to confidentiality and the sharing of information also deserve discussion so that misunderstanding can be avoided. Both the consultant and consultee must have clear understandings of the circumstances concerning when and what information may become appropriate for release and when it formerly was not. The issue of release of this information may need to be renegotiated during the consultation process. Most often it is the consultant who is in a position to destroy a consulting effort by revealing confidential information gained from the consultee or administration. If possible, information to be designated as confidential should be specified in the contract.

One common problem relates to the consultant's obligation to provide *complete* feedback. If the consultant discovers that something is seriously wrong in a system, or with an individual's performance, should the consultant always make it known? The answer often lies in weighing the relative importance of the consultation project as opposed to a desire not to alienate people in particular positions. The consultant must make it clear that he is not a "hired gun" and should be unwilling to accept the assignment of "going after people" and of criticizing or blaming them. However, if his job is to be thorough, it will normally have to include evaluation of the present system under consideration and feedback concerning those findings.

Limiting Scope and Defining Outcomes

In planning for consultation, Lombana (1979) suggests that the consultant limit the number of needs to be considered and set priorities. The contract should specify the needs to be met succinctly. Typically, the effort required to meet needs will be underestimated, and attempting to tackle too much will lead to problems later. Of the issues selected, the consultant and consultee must agree on an order of priority. Which needs are prerequisites to others? If it is determined that one need will have to be compromised to meet another, a priority order will be necessary to select the more important need.

It is recommended that the contract not stop at merely specifying needs. It should list goals and objectives that will be accomplished to meet the needs. It is suggested that objectives be observable and written in behavioral terms so that their accomplishment will be readily apparent to both the administration and consultee group at the end of the consultation project.

Conceptualizing the Contract

The development of a contract will be much easier if the consultant has a clear-cut perception of the nature of the services he intends to render. For example, in a school system, a consultant may at times work directly with a child and at other times work with a teacher, a group of teachers or the entire staff of a school with regard to the child. Caplan (1970) offers a fourfold system for classifying mental health consultation based on the kind of problem and the focus (client/program or consultee). He points out that, in practice, consultation is usually of a mixed type.

Caplan's description of consultation efforts is mentioned here as an organizational tool. It may help the consultant better conceptualize the nature of the work that he has before him. It is suggested that Caplan's approach be used as a basis for constructing goals and objectives for the consulting contract.

The four types of consultation described by Caplan are client-centered case consultation, consultee-centered case consultation, program-centered administration consultation and consultee-centered administrative consultation.

Client-centered case consultation occurs when a consultee seeks help with a particular case or group of cases and the consultant helps the consultee identify methods of dealing with the particular situation. Assuming that the consultant possesses relevant expertise, suggestions will be made following an evaluation of the situation by the consultant. For example, in a referral for a psychological evaluation, the school psychologist is asked to diagnose the difficulty and develop a plan of treatment. In this instance, the psychologist works directly with the child either to support or refute the problem as stated by the teacher. The teacher's perceptions should be sought, and the data should be discussed with the teacher. Possible solutions to the problem should be developed mutually, and recommendations should be offered in a nonthreatening way. Encouraging the teacher to assist in developing recommendations will improve chances that recommendations will be implemented. It is hoped that through this experience, the teacher will be better able to generate strategies for dealing with similar problems in the future.

In consultee-centered case consultation, a particular case or group of cases is again the presenting problem. However, in this type of consultation there is more of a collaborative problem-solving effort that aims at improving the consultee's problem-solving skills with similar cases in the future. The consultant is interested in exploring difficulties that the consultee is having in dealing with this situation. The consultee may be lacking in knowledge, skill, self-confidence or professional objectivity (Caplan, 1970). Wherever weaknesses are found, the consultant attempts to help the consultee find ways to overcome them and apply what he has learned to the particular situation as well as similar situations in the future.

This type of consultation may be appropriate when a teacher complains that a student's behavior is uncontrollable much of the time. Through observation and discussion with the teacher, the consultant may learn that the teacher lacks an understanding of effective behavior management techniques. The consultant does not work directly with the student, although a change in behavior is one objective. Changes in the teacher's behavior are the main focus of the intervention, which may include heightening the teacher's awareness of his difficulties and instruction in sound behavior management techniques. One intent is that the teacher will be able to generalize from what has been learned.

Program-centered administrative consultation involves helping a consultee with a particular program. In this type of consultation, the consultant helps the consultee develop or improve a program through an analysis of relevant issues, which leads to recommendations about how the administration might proceed. For example, a school system attempting to initiate a program for learning disabled youngsters may call upon a consultant with expertise in the organization and administration of such programs. After analyzing the situation, the consultant generates recommendations or suggestions about how best to proceed. By involving those concerned in the analysis and problem-solving tasks, it is hoped that the consultee will acquire knowledge and skills that will assist in dealing with similar issues in the future.

When the administrative consultation is consultee centered, the primary goal is to assist the consultee in identifying and remediating administrative problems that are occurring over a particular program instead of organizing and analyzing data about the program itself. For example, a group of administrators may be having difficulty establishing a desired program because they are not communicating effectively with one another. When the consultant recognizes such a difficulty, he attempts to develop strategies for improving the flow of information among the various administrators. By improving the communications, the group will be better able to achieve their objectives concerning the particular program as well as future programs. In this type of consultation, the details of the particular problem are less important than when the administrative consultation is program centered.

It is quite possible that a consultant may begin a consultation project with one particular goal in mind, e.g. client-centered case consultation. It may, however, become clear after working in the consultation relationship that consultee-centered case consultation is also dictated and that the consultant should redirect some of his efforts. It will be helpful if this type of redirection can be described as a possibility in the initial contract. This forethought will make necessary modification of the contract a much simpler task.

Evaluation of the Consultation Effort

An activity that must be provided for and needs to be outlined to the client during the planning stages is evaluation. Evaluation should measure the success of the program and how effectively the planned goals have been approached and met. This experience will usually communicate to those involved in hiring and working with the consultant that he did not know all the answers and was not able to correct all the program's problems, and that unforeseen circumstances and factors can confound the anticipated smooth execution of a plan. The clients should react to this experience and offer suggestions for more effective continuation of the procedures introduced. The consultant, on the other hand, must not feel threatened by a postconsultation evaluation. If the consultee's involvement in planning as well as implementing a program has been welcomed, and their opinions and skills as professionals respected, they will address the postconsultation evaluation task in a positive and professional manner and not use it to deny the talents or sincerity of the consultant. The program evaluation should not be viewed only as an end product but as a "dynamic process" (Trump, 1975, p. 17) that includes process and product evaluation to lead to additional programmatic changes in the future.

Follow-up

A good consultant will be available for some follow-up of his recommendations. Provisions for follow-up should be built into the consultant agreement. Not only does this serve to reinforce gains that have been made and provide an opportunity to correct difficulties, it helps maintain an open channel of communication between consultant and consultee, which may be important to possible consultation relationships in the future.

With the completion of the initial contract, the consultant should be ready to embark on the task of delivering the requested services. As with the contract, the entire process of consultation needs to be a dynamic process. There must be continual opportunities to renogotiate the contract and to change direction in midstream if necessary.

CRITICAL ISSUES IN THE IMPLEMENTATION OF SERVICES AND POTENTIAL FOR CONFLICT OF INTEREST

No matter how professional and thorough the consultant's description of his role and responsibilities, the consultation contract itself, and the consultant's preparation, there will be circumstances characteristic of each individual assignment that can interfere with effective consultation and that must be addressed. This section will deal with some potential areas of conflict for the consultant. Suggestions will be offered as to how the consultant can avoid certain difficulties or respond in an ethical, professional manner when they do occur.

Conflicts of Interest

Attention must be paid to potential conflicts of interest regarding the consultant's acceptance of remuneration, privileged communication, organizational loyalty and personal involvements. There can be no alliances, personal or professional, that will prevent a consultant from doing his job honestly and totally. As mentioned elsewhere, these issues are best dealt with before the onset of the actual consultation assignment. Such planning does not, however, preclude the emergence of serious problems.

The possibilities of conflict of interest and unethical behavior are issues that are not always clear. Obviously, if the consultant recommends that an organization buy goods or services from another organization from which he receives a secret "kickback," it is a clear case of unethical and possibly illegal behavior, but it is rarely so clear-cut. More often the consultant must be concerned with more mundane issues such as Am I charging for a service that the client should be receiving from me at no cost under other affiliations that I have? or Is the organization aware that it can receive these services free of charge elsewhere? The consultant must also take great pains to comply with protection of privacy, human rights and other codes and regulations. When in doubt, the consultant is advised to review the ethical code of his professional organization and, if still in doubt, discuss the question with one or more of his respected colleagues.

Controlling Consultant Personal Feelings

On a personal level, a consultant usually attempts to present himself as a credible, competent professional. If he takes pride in his work and puts forth time and energy toward his designated goals, his self-esteem (and professional reputation) will be enhanced by success. However, Fine et al. (1979) warn against the consultant's giving too much of himself emotionally because of either his personal stake in reaching his goals or his own belief in the value of his recommendations. There are many problems that can result from consultant overinvolvement.

One is the intentional, or inadvertent, revelation to clients that one has all or even most of the answers to their problems. An individual rarely does, and it is often destructive to have consultees believe so. Yet, this illusion can be conveyed by offering a solution too soon in the process, giving the impression that all circumstances are under control. Should relevant factors and complications have been overlooked, then the consultant will lose credibility, which may terminally damage the consultation effort. If the consultant responds with a "cure" without completing the evaluation and planning stages, or makes statements about how things are "supposed to be," he has taken ownership of the problem and will be held accountable for the project's success or failure (Fine et al., 1979). Having all the answers can also discourage enthusiastic participation by others because of the exclusive knowledge and responsibility claimed by the consultant.

The Need to Understand the Consultation Process

An individual may be very talented in his particular field, but he usually will not be an effective consultant if he has not been trained as a consultant. There is a special skill needed to be an effective consultant and to be able to deal with the problems that go beyond knowledge of content material (Brown et al., 1979; Lombana, 1979). For example, the mental health professional who accepts a consultation assignment must be cautious not to mistake consultation for psychotherapy. The consultant must not interpret meanings of statements, or the consultant's function must not be seen as a supervisory role, because it lacks ongoing supervisory contacts and the evaluation of employees that are part of a supervisor's job.

Medway (1979) implies that the consultation process is not a scientific process, does not follow experimental control procedures, and does not allow for control of the individual characteristics of the consultant or consultee. The consultant must be flexible enough to revise his plans to account for unexpected influences.

Martin (1978) advises that the consultant must adjust his style to either a one-to-one or to a group consultation depending on the situation. If working with clients in a group, the consultant must be able to foster group cohesion and coordination of efforts while maintaining each individual's confidentiality when necessary. The consultant will need to have acquired training in group work if he is to lead a group of unfamiliar people, perhaps resistant ones, to productive ends (Brown et al., 1979). Consultants who attempt to work with groups without the necessary group skills, or attempt to interact with a group in the same way one would with a single individual, are apt to encounter major difficulties.

The Need For Data

Another problem may arise when there is a lack of statistical records and follow-up data produced and kept during the course of consultation services (Medway, 1979). This often results in the inability of the consultant convincingly to communicate evaluation findings. Shaw (1977) recommends that a consultant maintain records with "hard" data to provide more understandable and accepted feedback during the course of and at the end of the consultation. While consultees and administration might be pleased with the viewpoints and opinions of the consultant, they will be more impressed with clear, well-interpreted data.

Generalization in the Consultation Process

Across all types of consultation, one of the consultant's goals should be to assist the consultee in learning ways of dealing with other similar situations. This requires a more generic approach after a problem-specific approach has been used. For example, the consultant may ask the consultee to problem-solve similar difficult situations and lend support to this process through encouragement and constructive criticism. Earlier in this chapter it was mentioned that training may be helpful in the initial stages of consultation. Later in the process, consultation must often be supplemented by training. This may include a demonstration or modeling of desired behaviors, experimental learning, critical discussion, practice and supervision. Training can result in a much more valuable consultation effort, since it may lessen the organizational need for continual consultation assistance. The consultee in one situation may apply his knowledge and skills as a consultant to others with similar problems (Kurpius, 1978).

If it is obvious that consultation will be a continuing need, then other approaches may be appropriate. There is something to be said for training consultees in being good consumers of consultative services as, for example, in training how properly to define and describe problems and how to ask appropriate questions about those problems. Consultees can learn to make judgments concerning when a problem is appropriate for consultative assistance and how most effectively to access that assistance. Within a school setting, for example, the encouragement and training that teachers receive as part of consultation tend to reduce significantly the number of referrals for services (Ritter, 1978). It may also lead to *earlier* detection and intervention (Chandler, 1980). Teachers tend to like the consultation model better for cases of moderate severity but feel more comfortable turning over the more difficult cases to another specialist (Gutkin et al., 1980). Typically, consultation is cheaper and more efficient for an organization than individual case study by an outside professional, and its use should be encouraged.

Hawthorne Effect

Meyers et al. (1978) suggest that the Hawthorne effect is in operation when a consultant appears on the scene in a given situation. The Hawthorne effect relates to the positive effect that normally occurs when individual problems are being closely attended to and the consultees feel that someone else really cares about their problems. When the consultant enters a new situation and begins to problem-solve and offer solutions, problems normally improve *simply because of this attention.* This initial improvement is something that the consultant can use to his advantage in accomplishing goals. The initial improvement will normally be viewed by the consultees as evidence of the consultant's skill and knowledge and will assist in gaining support for changing systems or consultee behavior. However, for the effect to continue, the consultant's efforts will need to lead toward more positive results. The consultant must be clearly aware that the Hawthorne effect will not last forever. It is simply a tool that is initially useful, but the success of the consultation effort cannot be solely dependent on incidental positive effects.

Consultation Report

Finally, the consultant should submit a report summarizing the goals of consultation and what was accomplished. A written report both adds closure to the process and assists in avoiding later misunderstandings about the process. It is recommended that a summary of the postconsultation evaluation also be contained in the report. The final written statement tends to improve the client's satisfaction, if for no other reason because it clearly demonstrates the consultant's continued concern regarding the problem and support of the organization after the original contract has been fulfilled.

CONCLUSION

It would be possible to explore many more issues under each of the sections presented in this chapter. The issues selected are examples of common concerns that arise in each area. Any major consultation project will raise a new issue or two or add a few twists to old issues. If consultants know the basic ground rules of consultation and approach the unexpected issues intelligently and cautiously, then their chances for success will be enhanced.

Each consultative situation will bring with it a set of individual personalities with whom to work, a system of procedures, rules, politics and ethics within which to work and any number of issues, known or unexpected, that the consultant must address to provide optimal service. While a consultant's preparation for effective consultation includes acquiring a wide variety of professional training experiences and conducting situation-specific planning, it also requires the ability to be sufficiently flexible to deal spontaneously with both content-related and unexpected humanistic occurrences.

Finally, it is of paramount importance to note that in and of itself, even vast knowledge of the consultation process will not assist in the delivery of appropriate services. This knowledge must be intelligently used. If a consultant, for example, chooses not to negotiate a contract at the beginning of the consultation process because it is inconvenient, then he has created certain liabilities for himself. More important, he has chosen to disregard the experience of many other consultants who have had their successes and failures and, as a result, have recommended that a contract format be adhered to.

There is already much repetition in the professional literature regarding the consultation process. Yet, there is a great deal that has not been explored and discussed. It is our hope that those with experience in the consultation process will share their experiences, thoughts and suggestions to create a more complete and useful literature than is now available. While we have learned much about the consultation process, there is still a great deal to be learned.

REFERENCES

1. Abidin, R.R. Operant behavioral consultations as conducted by masters and doctoral level psychologists in Virginia. *Journal of School Psychology*, 1977, *15*(3) 1225-28.

2. Brown, D., Wyne, M.D., Blackburn, J.E., & Powell, W. C. *Consultation: Strategy for improving education.* Boston: Allyn and Bacon, Inc., 1979.

3. Caplan, G. *The theory and practice of mental health consultation.* New York: Basic Books, 1970.

4. Chandler, L.A. Consultative services in the schools: A model. *Journal of School Psychology*, 1980, *18*(4), 399-402.

5. Cohen, L. D. *Consultation: A community mental health method.* Atlanta, Ga.: Southern Regional Education Board, 1964.

6. Fine, M.J., Grantham, V. L, & Wright, J. G. Personal variables that facilitate or impede consultation. *Psychology in the Schools*, 1979, *16*(4), 533-539.

7. French, J. R. P., Jr., & Raven, B. *The bases of social power.* In D. Cartwright (Ed.), *Studies in social power.* Ann Arbor: University of Michigan Institute of Social Research, 1959.

8. Golan, S., & Eisdorfer, C. *Handbook of community mental health.* New Jersey: Prentice-Hall, 1972.

9. Gutkin, T. B., Singer, J. H., & Brown, R. Teacher reactions to school-based consultation services: A multivariate analysis. *Journal of School Psychology*, 1980, *18*(2), 126-34.

10. Handler, L., Gerston, A., & Handler, B. Suggestions for improved psychologist-teacher communication. In J. Meyers, R. Martin, & I. Hyman (Eds.), *School consultation.* Springfield, Ill.: Charles C Thomas, 1977, 40-47.

11. Hartley, M. P. Consulting for change: Anatomy of an effort that failed. *Personnel & Guidance Journal*, 1979, *58*(1), 50-53.

12. Heller, K. Facilitative conditions for consultation with community agencies. *Personnel and Guidance Journal*, 1978, *56*(7), 419-423.

13. Kurpius, D. Consultation theory and process: In integrated model. *Personnel and Guidance Journal*, 1978, *56*(6), 335-338.

14. Lombana, J. H. A program-planning approach to teacher consultation. *The School Counselor*, 1979, *36*(3), 163-170.

15. Martin, R. Expert and referent power: A framework for understanding and maximizing consultation effectiveness. *Journal of School Psychology*, 1978, *16*(1), 49-55.

16. McGregor, D. *The human side of enterprise.* New York: McGraw-Hill, 1960.

17. Medway, F. J. How effective is school consultation? A review of recent research. *Journal of School Psychology*, 1979, *17*(3), 275-80.
18. Meyers, J., Pitt, N. W., Gaughan, E. T., Jr., & Friedman, M. P. A research model for consultation with teachers. *Journal of School Psychology*, 1978, *16*(2), 137-44.
19. Ritter, D. Effects of a school consultation program upon referral patterns of teachers. *Psychology in the Schools*, 1978, *15*(2), 239-243.
20. Rogawski, A. S. The Caplanian model. *Personnel & Guidance Journal*, 1978, *56*(6), 324-327.
21. Shaw, M. C. The development of counseling programs: Priorities, progress, and professionalism. *Personnel and Guidance Journal*, 1977, *55*, 339-345.
22. Trump, J. L. Illustrative models for evaluating school programs. *Journal of Research and Development in Education*, 1975, *8*, 16-31.

Chapter 6

ACCOUNTABILITY AND EVALUATION
IN CONSULTATION AND EDUCATION

DAVID R. RITTER

"**E**VERYBODY talks about it but nobody does it." For years, that phrase was synonymous with prevention. In reality, however, it is a far more apt description of evaluation.

The evaluation of mental health programs or services seems to be an anathema to practitioners in the field. It is an area of expertise in which the majority of practitioners feel less than competent, and to be done well, evaluation is a time-consuming and costly undertaking. Although expertise, time, and cost are significant factors, perhaps the greatest deterrent to effective evaluation of programs or services is the difficulty of translating research concepts and designs into applied settings. It is not so much the state of the art of applied evaluation that presents the barrier but the responses of audiences to the results of evaluation studies conducted within these applied settings. As most experienced community mental health center practitioners know, the rewards of evaluation are few. Evaluation studies conducted by the mental health centers tend to be criticized for their experimental designs, lack of comparison groups, and failure to control for possible intervening variables that could in and of themselves produce the eventual results. Having an evaluation study published in a professional journal is an equally arduous task. Having a manuscript rejected repeatedly does little to reaffirm the practitioner's motivation to evaluate services. Manuscript submissions again confront the issue of "pure" versus "applied" research. Criticism of practices for sub-ject selection alone leaves practitioners wide eyed in amazement: how does one randomly assign individuals to intervention groups when voluntary requests for a particular service or clinical issues do not permit randomization? It is fair to say that evaluation is, perhaps, the least rewarding of roles for the community mental health practitioner.

In recent years, the argument has been offered that evaluation is an absolute necessity if community mental health centers are to continue to receive funding from state or federal sources. From a community perspective, however, this poses a real catch-22. The community mental health center's first priority is to maintain ser-vices to the community to every extent possible. Decline in dollars means declining services. The problem is only compounded by such terms as accountability, validation or evaluation, as the com-munity mental health center is faced with reducing services to an even greater extent if it is to bear the staff time and cost of eval-uating those services. If a CMHC does make the difficult choice to curtail services further in favor of conducting evaluation, it is again catch-22. The expense associated with evaluation tends to increase the cost per unit of service, which, in turn, draws criticism from those same state or federal sources around the CMHC's "produc-tivity" and "efficiency." It is regrettable to say, but evaluation can be a "no win" situation.

Although there can be many problems and pitfalls associated with evaluation, this is not to say that it should not be seriously considered. There is risk in *not* evaluating programs and services, not the least of which is the tendency for service systems to be-come self-perpetuating, delivering the same services, which might have greater impact when provided in a slightly modified format. Indeed, some services may not have any significant benefit. Unless some attempt is given to evaluating programs and services, we can-not begin to ask the question of how services might be improved or address the more critical issue of whether they have value at all. We, as caregivers, *assume* that our services have value to those in-dividuals to whom they are provided. Whether or not they have value to us is not the issue; the real question is their level of value to those individuals who receive them. The question of service value is particularly cogent for Consultation and Education, as C&E's very survival hangs in the balance. Consultee dissatisfaction with services can lead to deterioration in what was formerly an effective working relationship, not to mention the monetary impact associated with the loss of a contract. Education or training programs that do not demonstrate their value go unenrolled. In the end, it is both the financial stability and credibility of Consultation and Education services that are affected.

PURPOSE OF EVALUATION

What is the purpose of an evaluation? For whom is an evaluation being conducted? What information is desired? The answers to these three questions will clarify the purpose of evaluation.

Understanding why an evaluation is to be undertaken is essential, as it sets the tone of the evaluation process, defines the extent of evaluation procedures, provides staff of the program to be reviewed with an understanding of the ground rules of the impact the evaluation might have upon the program, and defines the audiences for whom the results are intended. Purposes of evaluation can be many and varied. Evaluation might have the purpose of gathering information about community satisfaction with services, may seek to identify program strengths or weaknesses, may suggest areas of program modification, may be used to chart progress toward program goals, may seek to determine patterns of use of services, or may be designed to determine the impact of services through an assessment of outcome variables. Any of these purposes, either alone or in combination, would be appropriate in the evaluation of consultation or education services. Evaluation can be as simple as assessing the satisfaction of a consultee agency with services provided to them or as complex as assessing the long-term reduction of incidence of emotional disorders for a group of individuals participating in a program of primary prevention.

The extent to which evaluation will be conducted and the types of information that will be gathered will depend a great deal upon the audience to whom the evaluation results will be directed. Such audiences can either be internal or external to the CMHC. An internal audience might be program staff, administrators or perhaps even the governing board of the agency. External audiences would include individuals or agencies in the local community, legislators, funding sources, or federal or state monitoring agencies. As best possible, information to be gathered during evaluation should be responsive to those questions of greatest relevance to a particular audience. For example, while a state monitoring agency might be interested in a full profile of service use patterns within the CMHC's catchment area, such broad information might have little relevance to an individual community that is only interested in knowing how many of its own residents took advantage of services of the community mental health center and whether or not they were satisfied with those services. Similarly, if the intended audience is a funding source of a primary prevention program, it may be irrelevant to present information about participant satisfaction with the prevention program when the real question posed by the funding source is the program's prevention effectiveness. The matching of target audiences with appropriate information brings us to the issue of levels of evaluation.

TOPOLOGY OF LEVELS OF EVALUATION

In identifying information to be gathered from evaluation, it is helpful to conceptualize four levels of information. Each of these levels is quantitatively and qualitatively *different* from one another, and each level of information has its place and role in evaluation. Depending on the defined purpose of a particular evaluation, efforts are made to tap one or more levels of information. Essentially, the four levels of information include statistical information, satisfaction feedback, impact information, and outcome information.

Level 1 Evaluation — Statistical Information

The first level of evaluative information concerns itself with the gathering of statistical data. The method of evaluation is frequently a numerical count of various service variables such as hours of service, units of service, number of clients seen or individuals attending an educational program, numbers of consultations, numbers of training programs offered, etc. Statistical information is gathered in a very objective fashion. Information is obtained from daily activity sheets or from an agency's management information system and then is compiled into a profile of service delivery or use pattern. Level I Evaluation, the gathering of statistical information, is perhaps the most widely used evaluation procedure among community mental health centers. The information gathered is meaningful inasmuch as it describes *amounts* of services rendered to the community. However, Level I information cannot answer questions of satisfaction with services, the impact of services, or behavioral outcome as a result of participation in services. To answer these questions, one must move to a different level of information.

Level II Evaluation — Satisfaction Feedback

Level II evaluation has a primary focus on the question of satisfaction with services, with satisfaction defined as the subjective impression of the benefits accrued from a given service or program on the part of individuals who have been consumers of that service. Level II information is commonly gathered through questionnaire surveys or interview. Similar to the statistical information level, satisfaction feedback provides information that is directly relevant to program evaluation. The community mental health center is provided with meaningful information as to the center's image or acceptance within the community. Even though Level II information does not enhance knowledge about service impact or outcome, it does tap the pulse of the community's perception of the center and therefore is a most worthwhile endeavor.

Level III Evaluation — Impact

At Level III, evaluation begins to address the impact of programs or services upon individuals and groups. The most frequent evaluation approach is pretesting and posttesting on key variables such as an individual's gain in knowledge and information, understanding, awareness, competency, or coping skills. This level of evaluation has perhaps the greatest applicability to programs of an educational nature, as it seeks to assess skill gains on the part of participants. Both objective and subjective data are gathered: objective in the sense that gains in knowledge or skills are quantifiable through a pretest-posttest approach; subjective because one mode of obtaining information is from participant report. Within the clinical arena, an example of impact assessment would be reduction of symptomatology. Within an educational or preventive program, the assessed variables might be gains in parenting skills, assertive behavior or stress management techniques. For many community mental health services, Level III Evaluation of impact may well be an optimal level of program evaluation. Gains are able to be assessed over the short term rather than requiring more longitudinal investigation. While there are many advantages to program evaluation directed at the impact level, actual behavioral outcome information is still not obtained. A common error in the use of Level III Evaluation is that service agencies infer that gains in knowledge, awareness or skills become integrated into a person's behavioral style and are acted upon. This is a tenous inference at best. Level III only tells us the degree to which skills have been learned, not whether the skills have been effectively implemented.

Level IV Evaluation — Outcome

The assessment of behavioral outcome crosses the bridge from program evaluation to applied research. Level IV assesses actual behavioral change including change in a given person's daily functioning, behavioral style or actions. The change is both visible and quantifiable. The criterion are strictly objective. Methods of evaluation begin to use experimental and quasi-experimental designs in which individual behavior change is viewed over time or in which control group comparisons are employed. The evaluation design controls for intervening variables such as history or maturation in a controlled effort to document that behavioral change is due to the intervention program itself.

The evaluation of behavioral outcome is the true test of program effectiveness. It is a level to which evaluation should aspire as it truly addresses the question "Does a given program work?" Instead of the symptom reduction or skill gain focus of an impact level of evaluation, outcome addresses observable life situations such as employment, social relationships, school performance levels, the development of constructive leisure time alternatives or the maintenance of mental health and the ability to cope with normal life crises without the need to enter or reenter into treatment. Level IV Evaluation of Outcome requires a longer term commitment to the evaluation process, as outcome information is not necessarily immediately discernable but may require years of data gathering. For example, evaluating the question of whether a program targeted at children of mentally ill parents actually prevents children from themselves becoming mentally ill is a question that may not be answerable in five years of study, much less within five weeks or five months. Outcome evaluation is, however, that level of evaluation which contributes most meaningfully to the base of knowledge about program effectiveness and provides a true critical life variables assessment of whether programs work.

As previously noted, one should think of the four levels of evaluation as different from one another rather than one level necessarily being *better* than another. This is an important concept for Consultation and Education programs in particular, as information of a statistical or satisfaction nature may be far more valuable than would be any assessment of impact or outcome. Consultation and Education services are frequently oriented toward a particular segment of the community or even are consultee-specific; therefore, information about the amount of services provided and satisfaction with those services is often *the* primary evaluative information that is sought by the organizations or communities we serve. Fortunately, statistical and satisfaction information are also the easiest to be gathered, requiring little staff time or additional expense beyond that which would normally be invested in the particular consultation or education activity anyway. While the ideal might well be a Level IV evaluation of major outcome variables, the reality is that true outcome information is only rarely attained. Ironically, it is these major efforts at truly assessing outcome that are most open to criticism and challenge. From a cost-effectiveness point of view, a term that is becoming more and more familiar to C&E staff, the greatest evaluative benefit seems to derive from Level I to Level III information even though these levels do not truly provide what we need to know, that being whether a program really worked.

Table 6-I

LEVELS OF EVALUATION	I	II	III	IV
EVALUATION EMPHASIS	STATISTICAL	SATISFACTION	IMPACT	OUTCOME
MEASUREMENT AREA: In such areas as	Service Patterns e.g. hours; units; clients; programs; consultations	Service Satisfaction e.g. likes/dislikes; preferences;	Cognitive Gain e.g. knowledge; information; skills; awareness.	Behavioral Change e.g. actions, daily functioning; personal style.
MEASUREMENT EMPHASIS:	Numerical Counts of Service Variables;	Questionnaires; Feedback Forms;	Assessment of skill/Knowledge/Awareness gain	Assessment of visible behavioral change.
MEASUREMENT RELIABILITY:	Objective	Subjective	Subjective/Objective	Objective
MEASUREMENT METHODS:	Client/Consultation records; daily activity logs/timesheets;	Questionnaire/Survey of persons/agencies receiving service	Evaluation Design to Assess learning.	Evaluation Design to Assess integration of learning into action Longitudinal
Common Evaluation Methods:	Profile of Service , Utilization Patterns Computerized MIS G.A.S.	Client/Community Satisfaction Questionnaires G.A.S.	Evaluation/Research-Designs e.g. Pretest/Posttest	Evaluation/Research Designs e.g. Pretest/Posttest

THE EVALUATION PLAN

What design will be used in the evaluation? What evaluation measures will be employed to gather the desired information? What are the resources necessary to carry out the evaluation? These are the three primary questions for planning the evaluation.

Evaluation designs, whether experimental or quasi-experimental, form the structure of the evaluation plan. In considering design, the focus is on the areas of hypothesized outcome and the selection of the design iteself. Hypotheses are simply projections of desired outcomes that answer a typical sequence of "who, what, when, why and how." An example of a hypothesis statement might be as follows: It is hypothesized that significant change will be demonstrated in (what — skills or behavior), on the part of (whom — target group), when compared to (whom — comparison group), as a result of (why — the activity), as assessed (how — the measures). Hypotheses come into play when evaluation is focused on skills or outcome variables. A clear statement of hypotheses identifies the skill or competency to be developed, the participating target group, a comparison group (if any) against which gains of the target group will be measured, the activities or services to be provided, and the ways in which skill or competency gains will be measured. In many ways, hypotheses are akin to goal statements, and they can be formulated just as well for C&E activities as for direct client service activities. Two examples are in order, first for a consultation activity and second for an educational program. A school consultation service might embody a goal of assisting classroom teachers in more effectively managing the problem behavior of children. Thus, it would be hypothesized that significant change will be demonstrated in the *management of children's problem behavior*, on the part of *classroom teachers*, when compared to *teachers'* former management skills, as a result of *consultation* as assessed by *frequency with which children are sent to the principal's office for discipline*. A hypothesis of a course on parenting might be stated in the following manner: It is hypothesized that significant change will be demonstrated in *parent-child communication*, on the part of *parents*, when compared to *parents* who have not participated in a parenting course, as a result of *training in parent effectiveness* as assessed by *The Parent-Child Interaction Questionnaire.* As we can see from the above examples, the hypothesis statement is a clarification of the intent of a given service for a specific target group and how any skill gains will be measured. The hypothesis is, if you will, nothing more than an explicit behavioral objective.

Designs used for evaluation are really no more complex or confusing than are hypotheses, and if one is able to formulate a basic behavioral objective, then one is equally able to review and select an appropriate evaluation design. Rather than enter into a description of the full range of experimental of quasi-experimental designs, the reader is referred to Campbell and Stanley's (1963) monograph on the topic. For purposes of this chapter, only evaluation designs that seem to have the greatest relevance and use by Consultation and Education programs will be discussed.

Basically, there are two types of evaluation designs: those which compare individuals against themselves, and those which compare a group of individuals participating in a program or service against another group of individuals who do not receive the service. This latter group is commonly referred to as a control group. Evaluation designs are employed to answer one question: "Is there any reasonable evidence to suggest that a given program or service was at least partially responsible for change on the part of individuals participating in that program or receiving that service?" In evaluation, it is not sufficient simply to say that individuals changed, rather it must be demonstrated that this change was due in at least some way to their participation in a given program or service. This amounts to making some reasonable estimate of what changes might have occurred for persons had they not participated in a given program, comparing that estimate with actual changes on the part of participants, and then demonstrating that any differences between those figures are not attributed to simple chance or accident. The major differences among evaluation designs lie in how they go about forming those estimates and making these comparisons. Resultantly, evaluation designs use some kind of comparison group or, at the very least, some historical comparison of individuals against themselves. For Consultation and Education services, the most viable evaluation designs are either the group designs or the time-series designs.

The group designs have been found to be very useful to assess skills that have been learned as a result of participation in an educational program. Those who will be participating in the educational program complete some form of pretest measure (preferably an objective one) that assesses their level of skill prior to the program. Upon completion of the educational course, the participants again complete the same measure, this being the posttest. Differences between the two measures reflect the level of newly learned skills on the part of the participants. Since educational programs are typically of short duration, an assumption is made that any significant changes in skill levels would not have otherwise occurred for the group of individuals had they not participated in the educational program. However, from a research perspective, this is only an assumption. Nevertheless, the assumption can be made with reasonable validity, as long as there is only a brief time interval between testings. Since many community education programs are conducted on a day-long basis of perhaps an evening a week over six or eight weeks, the time interval is reasonable for the assumption to hold. Should an evaluator desire to be more certain that the changes in skill levels were, indeed, a result of the educational program itself, then some form of comparison group would be added to the design. Commonly called a control group, it consists of a number of individuals who are agreeable to completing the pretest and posttest measures but who will not be participating in the educational program itself. When data are analyzed, the gains made by the participant group as a whole are compared to the gains made by the control group, thus adding greater certainty that differences between these gain levels of the groups were a direct result of the educational program. Obviously, the greater the comparability among individuals in the intervention and control groups the more confidence one can place in the results.

Time series designs tend to be less widely used for evaluation purposes than do control group designs. Yet, these time series designs are perhaps the most tailored to an evaluation of preventive programs or consultation services. To evaluate effectively either consultation or preventive services, the evaluation must be conducted over longer periods of time than a simple pretest-posttest design allows. Time series designs allow for multiple measurements over time, both before involvement in a program to establish a baseline level of performance, at various times while the individuals are actually participating in the program or service, and subsequent to their participation to assess the impact of the service upon later behavior. The critical feature of this design is that assessments are made periodically and on a regular time interval basis such as weekly or monthly. The time series design provides information about the different levels of performance before, during and after the intervention.

As with the group designs, time series designs can be used either for a single group of individuals or as a multiple time series format that compares the group participating in the service with another comparable group that has not participated. In either case, there is an expectation for behavioral change on the part of participants at or about the time that the service or program is initiated, and there is an expectation that behavior after a service has begun to be delivered will differ from behavior prior to individuals having the opportunity to receive that service.

Let us use an organizational consultation example to describe further the time series design:

A local industry approaches its community mental health center with a request for organizational development consultation to help the industry develop an Employee Assistance Program. Specific needs of the industry are to develop organizational procedures within its personnel department that can facilitate employees obtaining treatment services that may be necessary for the maintenance of their on-the-job functioning and productivity, to train front-line supervisors in the early identification of troubled employees, and to develop a network of referral agreements whereby prompt and confidential services can be provided for employees in need. To determine the impact of any new Employee Assistance Program, it is necessary to evaluate outcome. A time series design is ideal for this type of evaluation project. The design will assess the impact of a change in organizational policy, in this case the assistance program, across such variables as employees' loss of productivity while on the job, use of sick time and employee turnover.

The new Employee Assistance Program is scheduled to begin its operation six months in the future. Initially, at a three-month interval and at the six-month interval, the industry's loss of employee productive time, use of sick time and rate of employee turnover are measured to gather a baseline on these main variables. The Employee Assistance Program is implemented at its six month target date, and three months later, six months later and nine months later the rate of lost employee productive time, use of sick time and employee turnover are again calculated. The impact of the Assistance Program would be demonstrated based upon a difference in the key variables before and after the implementation of the program. It would be expected that the program would increase the productive function of employees on the job while at the same time decreasing use of sick time and reducing the rate of employee turnover. As long as the Employee Assistance Program was the only major organizational change during this period, then changes in employee productivity and turnover would be attributed to the implementation of the program. It is assumed that without such a program the losses of productive time and rate of employee turnover during the baseline period would continue to exist.

As one can see from the above example, the time series design is particularly useful to evaluate changes in organizational practices or the introduction of a new program. As for statistical analyses, they require neither elaborate analyses nor a computer. A simple t-test of baseline versus postprogram implementation will suffice. However, there is one caution that is offered around the interpretation of baseline versus postprogram implementation data. The introduction of any new practice or program may, in and of itself, result in a temporary or transitional change in the levels of some variables. To be cautious, there should be very significant and ongoing change in the variables being evaluated if one is to interpret the program as being effective.

The questions of evaluation measures and resources needed to conduct the evaluation are intertwined. Obviously, the choice of assessment measures to be used in evaluation will depend on the expertise of the individuals who will be administering the measures and the time commitment of these individuals. Both the purchase price of the measures themselves and the staff time required translate into an outlay of money. Therefore, the issue of resources and instrumentation is addressed prior to the actual conduct of the evaluation.

The types of measures to be used will depend on the level of information that is sought, whether statistical, satisfaction, impact or outcome. It will also depend on the variables to be measured. While a standardized instrument may be available to assess attitudes, knowledge or behaviors, it may be necessary to create one's own instrument, such as a questionnaire, to measure satisfaction or certain life variables such as employment. Measures can be either norm referenced or criterion referenced, but regardless of the choice of instrumentation, the measures themselves should be able to provide both reliable and valid assessments of the variables that are to be measured. Within the realm of C&E, available measures are far less sophisticated or standardized than those which might be used to assess clinical outcome. While this may pose some hindrance to evaluation of consultation or education approaches, it should not be seen as a barrier that is insurmountable.

There are a few caveats that are offered for the actual conduct of the evaluation. By far, questions of staff time and scheduling are of the greatest concern. It is absolutely necessary for an individual to be assigned the overall responsibility for managing or coordinating the evaluation. This person would not only be involved in the planning of the evaluation but would also oversee the evaluation process itself, including the gathering of information, the analysis of data and the compilation of a summary report. Staff who actually conduct the evaluation must be clear in their responsibilities. Scheduling must be strictly adhered to in the collection of information, especially if a time series design is being employed. What will be administered, to whom, by what staff persons and at what times during the year are critical questions. How data will be collected and where it will be compiled and stored are equally important, for the loss of already collected data can be a major blow to an evaluation project.

ANALYSIS OF INFORMATION AND REPORTING OF RESULTS

How will data be analyzed? To whom and in what format will it be disseminated? These are the two questions for the final aspect of the evaluation process.

Data analysis, by necessity, will have to remain rather simple unless the community mental health center is in some way affiliated with a college or university and can tap the expertise and/or computer capabilities of such an institution. Clearly, a detailed presentation of statistical analysis procedures is beyond the scope of this chapter, and the reader is referred to one of the many texts that are available today on the subject.

For the basic group of time series designs that have been discussed, some rather simple statistical procedures can readily serve in data analysis. For designs involving pretests and posttests, a correlated t-test to assess the significant difference between pretest and posttest means can be employed. For those designs which employ a control group, a comparison of pretest-posttest gain scores of each group can also be performed through the use of the t-test, although admittedly this procedure is not the most powerful of statistical analysis methods. For the time-series designs, either with or without comparison groups, data analysis can consist of a determination of the significant differences between baseline levels and postintervention levels. Time series designs also lend themselves to visual and graphic representation of outcomes. Recalling the example of the Employee Assistance Program developed by a local industry, the following graphic representation would clearly show the impact of the program on, for example, the variable of employee turnover:

The impact of the program is demonstrated by the change in slope at the point of the implementation of the program, called the point of intercept. Equally important is the representation of the continuing reduction in employee turnover.

Practically speaking, there are a number of evaluation studies that fall under the purview of C&E for which a statistical approach to data analysis is not required. Perhaps the most obvious of these are evaluations of service satisfaction, whether on the part of consultees or individuals who have participated in a community education or training program. Such information on satisfaction with services is typically translated into percentages of individuals who are satisfied or dissatisfied with services, or similarly, the percentages of individuals who have found a certain service to be beneficial to them. While such data compilation procedures are rudimentary, the use of visual graphics, even a bar graph reflecting percentage of satisfaction, can serve to make the data analysis *look* more sophisticated than it actually is. The visual mode of presentation of information also links itself to greater understanding on the part of target audiences, not to mention its carrying a greater impact.

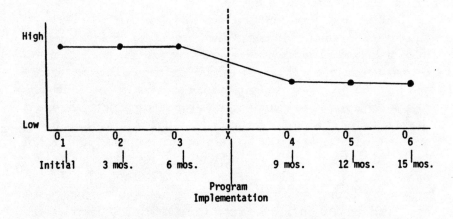

As one plans the analysis of information and the ways it will be recorded, it is essential to refer again to the question of target audience for whom the evaluation is intended. The choice of target audience will affect the way information is presented and results are reported, for example the use of technical versus laymen's language, whether or not results are being used to justify continued funding of a given program, whether the purpose of the evaluation was to demonstrate program efficacy, or whether its intent was simply to provide information about the types and levels of services provided and individual satisfaction with the services. The dissemination plan should address in detail to whom the results will be reported, by whom they will be presented and the method in which they will be shared, which may include a printed document, a slide-sound presentation, or an in-person presentation. If the evaluation study is to be conducted over a long period of time, then a decision will need to be made on the timing of interim reports that can demonstrate progress to date. For C&E it is likely that there would be three primary audiences for evaluation results. The first audience would be an internal one, that being staff of the C&E program itself. A few visual graphics and a presentation by the person conducting the evaluation would seem to suffice in sharing evaluation results with staff. A second common audience for C&E would be the community itself, perhaps in the form of a local town governing body. A brief written summary with a few tables would be the likely format and would prove quite worthwhile as an adjunct to any presentation seeking town contribution or funding of community services of the mental health center. The third likely audience, and regrettably one that seems to be diminishing for C&E, is that of local, state and federal funding agencies who have supported a particular program with the expectation that an evaluation of program impact was conducted. These presentations usually take the form of interim or final reports that incorporate a full description of the program, services that have been delivered under it, and the evaluation results. Reports to funding or monitoring agencies tend to be more comprehensive in their scope and are frequently written in the jargon of the profession, always of course, "spicing-in" those words or phrases which happen to be the key words of the times. Funding or monitoring agencies seem to thrive on computerlike language, and reports filled with terminology such as "input," "output," "linkage," "interface," etc. seem to be well received. Similar language, however, does little to enhance the humanistic image of the mental health center on the part of the general community.

Overall, a useful guideline for C&E would be to evaluate one service/program per year. Since C&E will be involved in far more than a single service, the effect will be that program evaluation is rotated annually, with each service or program being evaluated periodically. A rotating system permits evaluation resources to be maximized each year, since they are directed toward a single evaluation effort rather than spread among multiple evaluation projects. Depending upon the particular service to be evaluated in a given year, it becomes a natural event that the levels of information to be gathered, the target audiences for evaluation, and the complexity of the evaluation procedures will vary over time. Evaluation also becomes an ongoing process for the Consultation and Education program and affords a greater level of comfort for staff as evaluation becomes common-place.

ALTERNATIVE EVALUATION APPROACHES

In addition to experimental or quasi-experimental evaluation, there are a few other evaluation approaches that are applicable for C&E. Goal Attainment Scaling and Performance Contracting are but two of these alternatives.

Goal Attainment Scaling

The Goal Attainment Scaling (GAS) technique was developed by Kiresuk and Sherman (1973) through their work at the Hennepin County Mental Health Service in Minneapolis, Minnesota. As such, it is one of the few evaluation methods developed *by* mental health professionals *for* mental health professionals. In its original form, GAS was used to evaluate individual client treatment outcomes ranging from the least favorable treatment outcome to the most favorable outcome. Despite this original GAS focus toward assessing the impact of individual client treatment, the technique carries the potential for much broader application in the area of evaluation. In recent years, Goal Attainment Scaling has been widely used for the evaluation of educational programs (Carr, 1979; Cooper, Epperley, Forrer & Inge, 1977; Keelin, 1977) and a number of nonclinical community mental health approaches (Cline, Rouzer & Bransford, 1973; Kaplan & Smith, 1977; Kiresuk & Lund, 1975).

The GAS method uses a matrix format with goals on one axis and possible levels of attainment on the other axis. Typically, levels of attainment are described across a five-point Likert scale of possible outcomes, although a three-point scale can be used instead. Regardless of whether a five-point or a three-point scale is selected, the crucial variable is that the described attainment levels are significantly different from one another in order that adequate discrimination can be made between possible outcomes. The expected level of attainment will always fall at the midpoint of the rating scale's numerical continuum.

An attractive feature of the GAS method is that it does not require a great deal of sophistication in research knowledge or experience. Instead, the method can be used by any individual who is able to define clear program or service goals and possible outcomes. Those individuals whose forté is program evaluation can go beyond the basic GAS procedure by using an elaborate scoring system in which relative weights are assigned to each goal area, raw scores are translated to T scores and overall goal attainment change scores are calculated (see Hagedorn, Beck, Neubert & Werlin, 1976).

In relationship to the previously discussed topic of levels of evaluation, Goal Attainment Scaling can be a particularly useful procedure to gather Level I — Statistical and Level II — Satisfaction information. The procedure also has direct applicability to *process* evaluation and can serve as a procedure through which goals and objectives of program development or implementation are assessed. In community mental health centers where staff work under a management-by-objectives (MBO) agreement, Goal Attainment Scaling can be linked with that MBO contract and can serve as a method of performance evaluation. When used as a method of individual performance, however, it is extremely important that goals identified in the attainment scale be mutually determined by the persons involved. This insures agreement on established goals and clear identification of the expectations for level of attainment and increases the likelihood of cooperation toward achieving the goals.

The most significant drawbacks to the GAS method include its relative lack of applicability of Level III — Impact and Level IV — Outcome areas and the potential for bias entering into the actual establishment of goals and levels of attainment. A GAS evaluation of impact or outcome variables can all too readily be hindered by the often subjective nature of the defined attainment levels. Clearly, the evaluation of service impact or outcome requires strong objective data. Bias can come into play in the establishment of possible attainment levels. When GAS is used for the purposes of program evaluation, the risk of bias is enhanced if the individual establishing the goals and levels of attainment is also the individual who is responsible for the program being evaluated. The main issue is the establishment of reasonable and realistic expectations of attainment. Should a program manager wish to protect a program, in effect guarantee favorable outcome, all that needs to occur is a downward adjustment of attainment expectations. At the extreme, this would involve a typically average level of attainment being transformed into the most favorable attainment. Conversely, GAS can be abused in the opposite manner. Should a manager desire to modify or perhaps eliminate a given program, it would be a simple matter of modifying the attainment continuum so that the most favorable outcome became the average level of attainment. In an era of ever-increasing emphasis on accountability and service justification, there is greater risk of GAS being used to justify service systems and thereby perpetuate their existence.

Let us look at a sample Goal Attainment Scale using the case of a school-based prevention program. Let us assume that this program is just beginning its implementation stage and that the focus of the program is an affective education curriculum being pilot tested within a school district. Table 6-II portrays the Goal Attainment Scale, having five program goals each with its continuum of attainment from the most unfavorable to the most favorable results. The possible levels of attainment have been established in a manner appropriate to the GAS procedure, with the average expectation falling at midpoint on the continuum. This average expectation level is thought to be the most likely outcome by the end of the program's implementation year. The average expectation would include program implementation in three of the six elementary schools in the district; program satisfaction on the part of 80 percent of the teachers whose classrooms receive the affective education curriculum; that these same teachers who have been satisfied will continue the programs in their classrooms; that a tight financial situation carries the likelihood of an 80 percent level of continuation funding; and that an evaluation procedure will be conducted for the program. In developing the attainment continuum, the extremes of program failure or program success well beyond reasonable expectations are established. Clearly, these most unfavorable and most favorable ends of the continuum are truly extremes, and it is quite unlikely that either will occur.

Table 6-II
GOAL ATTAINMENT SCALE: SCHOOL AFFECTIVE
EDUCATION PROGRAM

GOALS	OUTCOMES				
	1 *Least* *Favorable*	2	3 *Average* *Expected*	4	5 *Most* *Favorable*
PROGRAM IMPLEMENTATION	no schools implement program	2 of 6 schools implement	3 of 6 schools implement	4 of 6 schools implement	all schools implement program
PROGRAM SATISFACTION	0 % teachers satisfied	50 % teachers satisfied	80 % teachers satisfied	90 % teachers satisfied	100 % teachers satisfied
PROGRAM CONTINUATION	no schools continue program	2 of 6 continue program	3 of 6 continue program	4 of 6 continue program	all schools continue program
PROGRAM FUNDING	funding ended	50 % funding continues	80 % funding continues	full funding continues	funding in excess of past year
PROGRAM EVALUATION	no evaluation conducted	–	evaluation conducted completely	–	evaluation exceeds original plan

Table 6-III presents a second Goal Attainment Scale for the same school-based prevention program. Let us assume that the same expectations as described in the former GAS are reasonable, but there are some other variables that interfere with an honest GAS. These variables might be that the coordinator of the affective education program is heavily invested in the program being successful, that for political or public image purposes the program needs to succeed, or that continued funding for the program by the school district demands that positive results be attained. Then we have a very different GAS. Successful outcome across the five goal areas is guaranteed by moving the average expected level of attainment to the position of most favorable level of attainment. By modifying the criteria on the GAS attainment continuum, the identical program experience at the end of the year can be rated as achieving either average attainment or the most favorable attainment possible.

Table 6-III
GOAL ATTAINMENT SCALE: BIASED EVALUATION
OF SCHOOL AFFECTIVE EDUCATION PROGRAM

GOALS	OUTCOMES				
	1 Least Favorable	2	3 Average Expected	4	5 Most Favorable
PROGRAM IMPLEMENTATION	no schools implement program	–	1 of 6 schools implement	2 of 6 schools implement	3 of 6 schools implement
PROGRAM SATISFACTION	0 % teachers satisfied	20 % teachers satisfied	40 % teachers satisfied	60 % teachers satisfied	80 % teachers satisfied
PROGRAM CONTINUATION	no schools continue program	–	1 of 6 schools continue	2 of 6 schools continue	3 of 6 schools continue
PROGRAM FUNDING	funding ended	20 % funding continues	40 % funding continues	60 % funding continues	80 % funding continues
PROGRAM EVALUATION	no evaluation conducted	–	partial evaluation conducted	–	complete evaluation conducted

Although the problem of bias is a very real issue, a concept that may have equal implications in the use of Goal Attainment Scaling is the concept of "average" outcome. For those individuals involved in program evaluation, the concept "average" carries statistical connotations of mean, median or mode. Average has statistical meaning; it is the concept that denotes the midpoint across a normal distribution. For many individuals, however, the concept of "average" carries negative connotations. Average does not convey an impression of success. It can be interpreted as mediocracy. Average connotes adequacy but certainly not greatness. However, where GAS is concerned, average has a very different meaning. It denotes full goal attainment; it describes a level of significant success. Indeed, for those who wish to use Goal Attainment Scaling as a method of evaluation, it may be advantageous to replace the term "average expectation" with "full expectation." For the evaluator this may be nothing more than a game of semantics. For external audiences or funding sources, however, the change of wording may make the difference between a program's continuation and its demise.

Performance Contracting

The practice of performance contracting is beginning to come into its own as a method of evaluation. It is a procedure that focuses primarily on the evaluation of staff performance, although practically speaking the performance of staff bears a direct relationship to the performance of a particular program or service.

Performance contracting is an outgrowth of a system of management by objectives (MBO), through which specific behavioral outcomes are established with staff against which annual performance is evaluated. Many community mental health centers have used and continue to use MBO systems with their staff, and those familiar with an MBO approach can easily adopt performance contracts. Perhaps the major factor that differentiates one approach from another is that performance contracting is linked directly with levels of staff reimbursement or salary. In doing so, there is a tangible monetary benefit for staff meeting or exceeding their performance contracts and the specific objectives contained therein. Staffs' levels of remuneration become variable rather than fixed, and income itself becomes a strong motivator and reinforcer that encourages both efficient use of time and high quality services. This variable nature of salary expense does pose an interesting challenge for a program administrator, because if performance contracting is to work successfully the budget of the program itself must be flexible.

The performance contract represents a mutual agreement between a staff member and the program administrator in specifying specific areas of functioning and expected areas of performance. Staff remuneration is tied to those objectives and performance criteria, either by a percentage of salary being attached to each function and outcome or through specific blocks of service time being defined for each function and this time being reimbursed at a certain hourly wage. For instance, a performance function of a community educator might be the development of a three-part series of educational programs for the community. The specifics of the program plan are defined, including the number of programs to be developed and offered and the target dates for implementation. It is estimated that 20 percent of the community educator's time will be devoted to this endeavor and, therefore, an amount corresponding to 20 percent of salary is attached to this objective. If the performance objective is fully met, then the full level of reimbursement is earned. Partial attainment of a performance objective yields only partial reimbursement of the salary amount attached to that objective. Conversely, attainment at a level beyond that expected, either as a result of meeting the objective in advance of time lines or developing a program that receives tremendous response from the community, warrants a level of remuneration greater than that which would have been normally received. This additional compensation might be in the form of a salary bonus, additional vacation time, attendance at a conference, or any number of other possibilities that are valued by the staff person as long as they are mutually agreed upon at the time of performance contracting. This incentive system is the key to performance contracting, for without it the system involves consequences for performance failures but fails to offer rewards for exceptional performance. A second example of a performance contract, this time using the hourly wage concept of reimbursement, would be a C&E staff member providing consultation to a local agency under contract. The contract specifies four hours of consultation per week, and therefore, this becomes the expected service performance level. The hourly reimbursement to the staff person under the performance contract would be a sum that allows for both the direct service time as well as supportive time needed for travel, consultation records, etc. The consultant is reimbursed based upon the direct hours of service provided, the expectation being that the number of hours specified in the consultation contract are delivered. It is recognized that this example still lacks an incentive component, because the consultant's maximum hours cannot exceed the maximum time specified in the contract. Thus, it becomes necessary to identify an alternative incentive, the most likely being service satisfaction. The performance contract would include an agreement to assess consultee satisfaction at midyear and at the end of the year, based upon a questionnaire that would seek information on the benefits of consultation as perceived by the consultees themselves. As with the former example, the form of the incentive is specified in the performance contract as is the level of consultee satisfaction that would meet the incentive criteria.

Performance contracts and their accompanying incentive aspects can be used to promote the development of new programs or services as well. Performance goals and incentives can be used to motivate and reward staff entreprenurial efforts, such as the attainment of a new contract for services, the expansion of an existing contract or the development of a new service program that receives positive response from the community. With some thought and creativity, the full and sometimes diverse functions of a staff member can be incorporated into a performance contract, and the motivating factors can range from monetary to intangible, from dollars to flextime. The performance contract system derives benefits for both the C&E program and its staff; the former benefiting from a high level of staff functioning, its accompanying positive public image and potential for the development of increased sources of income; and the latter because, in some form, staff are working for themselves as well as the program.

From an evaluation perspective, performance contracting lends itself to the gathering of information across all four levels: statistical, satisfaction, impact and outcome. Performance contracts are also cost-effective. They serve to maximize the percentage of staff time devoted to direct services, explicitly link costs with specific functions or services of the C&E program and enhance overall fiscal and programmatic accountability. As one can see, there are many advantages to a performance contract system. Yet, there are some potential disadvantages and pitfalls that should not be overlooked. It is imperative that the roles and functions of staff be stated in behavioral terms, that the criteria goals be clearly understood, and that the completed performance contract be mutually agreed to and signed by both the staff person and the C&E director. Of equal concern are the performance goals and objectives themselves. They must be designed to challenge the staff person but at the same time need to be realistically established so that there is ample room for success as well as possibilities of failure.

Performance contracts whose goals, objectives and evaluative criteria are established at an unrealistically high level will, in the end, impede a staff member's functioning and may even throw the C&E program itself into turmoil. As anyone familiar with basic learning and behavioral theory knows, reward systems only begin to function effectively when individuals participating in the system recognize that it is a fair and just paradigm and that successful attainment of targets is possible.

Some final caveats about performance contracting deal with salary or wage levels and incentives. Although it is quite possible for staff to set their own desired salary levels, this can only be done by staff modifying the amount of their work. Reimbursement rates themselves, whether salary dollars attached to a specific performance objective or defined hourly reimbursement, are set by the C&E director and are not negotiable. Even within this context certain parameters need to be set on how little or how much time staff are allowed to work. A staff person seeking greater income can fall into the trap of being overly optimistic in establishing a work load and run the risk of being overextended. At evaluation time, that staff person may have failed to meet any performance criteria, not because of lack of effort, but due to excessive work demands. The C&E director plays the role of balancer at the time performance contracts are written, adjusting work loads and performance objectives as best possible to coincide with the staff person's desires and the program's needs. This balancing role also comes into play for staff incentives. It *is* preferable for staff to identify those incentives which are truly of value to them. Yet, the C&E director retains veto power over those incentives which are deemed to be unreasonable or are simply unable to be provided due to resource limitations of the C&E department. It is also necessary to weigh incentives against the level of effort and performance objective to which they are attached so that equity prevails. Otherwise, staff would be inordinately rewarded at too high or too low a level for their accomplishments.

Whenever possible, performance contracts should be written for an entire year and should address each role and function of the staff person. Contracts should be individualized for staff so that staff work toward a specific standard or goal rather than compete against one another, a situation that can occur under a group contract. Performance contracting is not intended to create staff competition, and it is inappropriate to establish one major incentive that can only be attained by a single staff member — the person who excels the greatest. When used appropriately, performance contracting can be a strong motivator for staff, one that has benefit for the individual and the C&E program alike. It is also a clear and objective method of staff evaluation.

REFERENCES

Campbell, D., & Stanley, J. Experimental and quasi-experimental designs for research. In N. Gage (Ed.), *Handbook of research on teaching,* Chicago: Rand McNally & Company, 1963.

Carr, R. Goal attainment scaling as a useful tool for evaluating progress in special education. *Exceptional Children,* 1979, *46*(2), 88-95.

Cline, D., Rouzer, D., & Bransford, D. Goal attainment scaling for a method of evaluating mental health programs. *American Journal of Psychiatry,* *1973, 130*(1), 105-108.

Cooper, J., Epperley, J., Forrer, S., & Inge, J. Goal attainment scaling: A useful program evaluation tool. *Journal of College Student Personnel,* 1977, *18,* 522.

Hagedorn, H., Beck, K., Neubert, S., & Werlin, S. *A working manual of simple program evaluation techniques for community mental health centers* (No. 017-024-00539-8) Washington, D.C.: U.S. Government Printing Office, 1976.

Kaplan, J., & Smith, W. The use of attainment scaling in the evaluation of a regional mental health program. *Community Mental Health Journal,* 1977, *13*(2), 188-193.

Keelin, P. Goal attainment scaling and the elementary school counselor. *Elementary School Guidance Counseling,* 1977, *12*(2), 89-95.

Kiresuk, T., & Lund, S. Process and outcome measurement using goal attainment scaling. In J. Zusman & C. Wurster (Eds.), *Program evaluation, alcohol, drug abuse, and mental health services.* Lexington, Massachusetts: Lexington Books, 1975.

Kiresuk, T. & Sherman, R. Goal attainment scaling: A general method for evaluating comprehensive community mental health programs. *Community Mental Health Journal,* 1968, *4,* 443-453.

Wilson, N., Mumpower, J. Automated evaluation of goal attainment ratings. *Hospital and Community Psychiatry,* 1975, *26,* 163-164.

Chapter 7

PREVENTION IN COMMUNITY MENTAL HEALTH

CAROLYN F. SWIFT

INTRODUCTION

THE fascination of folk tales is that they embody the collective wisdom of the human condition. Screened through the scholarship of prevention, their messages comprise a respectable list of accepted prevention strategies. The ant already knew what the grasshopper had to learn: laying by summer grain staves off winter hunger. Anticipatory guidance also saved the third pig of the fabled trio, whose preference for bricks over straw turned out to be an effective wolf deterrent. Hansel and Gretel had the right idea in planning ahead, but even a cursory impact study would have demonstrated the vulnerability of bread crumbs to environmental influences. If these tales don't teach children how to prevent starvation, annihilation and abandonment, at least they sanction the value — through intervention and repetition — of making preventive efforts.

The persuasiveness of prevention lies in its axiomatic simplicity. Who can oppose the proposition that it's better to prevent dysfunction than to wait for it to occur and then treat it? Critics, however, read vagueness for simplicity and pronounce the concept too broad to be meaningful. Almost any behavior, after all, can be explained as preventive: eating prevents hunger, bathing prevents filth, exercise prevents atrophy, paying the rent prevents eviction, and so on. Prevention in this context means little more than behavior having purpose. Most of us act, individually or in groups, either to prevent or promote something, and pointing this out does little to advance science. Kessler and Albee (1975), in their classic review of the field, note this problem:

> During this past year we found ourselves constantly writing references and ideas on scraps of paper and emptying our pockets each day of notes on the primary prevention relevance of childrens' group homes, titanium paint, parent-effectiveness-training, consciousness raising, Zoom, Sesame Street, the guaranteed annual wage, legalized abortion, school integration, limits on international cartels, unpolished rice, free prenatal clinics, antipollution laws, a yogurt and vegetable diet, free VD clinics, and a host of other topics. Nearly everything, it appears, has implications for primary prevention, for reducing emotional disturbance, for strengthening and fostering mental health. (P. 560)

DEFINITION

The task is one delimiting the field. Prevention in community mental health is concerned with behavior. Nonbehavioral events such as natural disasters are of interest only as they have an impact on behavior. The history of prevention over the last two decades documents attempts to operationalize the term. An early attempt at clarification, borrowed from the field of public health, identified three levels of prevention — primary, secondary and tertiary. In this schema, primary prevention refers to the reduction of new cases of behavioral dysfunction in a population (incidence); secondary prevention refers to the reduction of the duration of dysfunction through early case finding and treatment; and tertiary prevention refers to attempts to minimize the chronic or permanent damage associated with dysfunction. The three levels correspond roughly to the lay concepts of prevention, treatment and rehabilitation. Anthony (1977) puts it succinctly: The three levels prevent "nothing from becoming something, mild disorder from becoming moderate, and moderate disorder from becoming severe."

Theoretical disagreements about classifying preventive interventions are common. The major controversy involves the distinction between primary and secondary prevention. Efforts at primary prevention are directed to persons who do not have the disorder being prevented. By preventing new cases from developing (reducing incidence), the total number of persons in the population having the disorder (prevalence) is also reduced. Efforts at secondary prevention, in contrast, are directed to persons who already have the disorder. Through early case finding and treatment, it is expected that the duration of the disorder will be reduced, thus reducing prevalence. Much of the prevention research published as primary is more accurately classified as secondary (Cowen, 1980), since the population targeted has often been selected on the basis of some deficit that is a part of the condition to be prevented.

The conceptual fuzziness in differentiating between primary and secondary prevention is rooted in two sources. The first is a misunderstanding of the identified target population. While it is a contradiction in terms to attempt to implement primary prevention programs aimed at reducing crime in a population of felons, it *is* possible to implement primary prevention programs aimed at reducing the incidence of schizophrenia, depression or other behavioral disorders that do not already exist for this population. A population that suffers some specified deficit can appropriately be targeted for primary prevention programs aimed at *other* deficits. Thus, attempts to reduce the incidence of substance abuse among the physically disabled, depression for the retarded or child abuse on the part of the unemployed are all legitimately classified as primary prevention activities. The chronic population is most often overlooked on the mistaken grounds that since they already exhibit dysfunction on one dimension, they are ineligible for primary preventive efforts on any other dimension. Reflection on the range of physical, psychological and social deficits found in a random population — heart disease, hypertension, acne, depression, insomnia, claustrophobia, divorce, unemployment, poverty, to name a few — reveals the error of this type of reasoning. The search for a pure (deficit free) population for primary prevention efforts is not only wrong but doomed, since each of us, figuratively speaking, carries an idiosyncratic set of physical, psychological and social warts. It is reasonable, then, to insist that the population targeted be free of the deficit condition being prevented, but not of other deficits, so as to classify prevention efforts as primary.

The second source of confusion between primary and secondary prevention has to do with the concept of risk. In general, persons are considered to be at risk if they are members of a group in which the incidence of a specified disorder is above the base rates for that disorder in the population (Vance, 1977). For example, children of schizophrenics are at a higher risk for developing this disorder than other children; the probability is 10 percent for children with one schizophrenic parent, compared with 1 percent for children without schizophrenic parents.

Whereas secondary prevention screens to detect disorders early, primary prevention, through prospective risk research, screens to detect dispositional factors associated with the subsequent development of disorders. Confusion results from the overlap between dispositional factors and incipient signs of the disorder to be prevented. Most definitions of risk do not exclude — and some explicitly include — the possibility that components of the potential disorder already exist in persons assigned risk status. As Bell and Pearl have stated, ". . .the concept of risk implies the ability to identify groups of individuals who, on the average, do not now show a disorder, *or only show components of the disorder,* but who have statistically significant likelihood of showing the disorder in full form at a later time, in comparison with a non-risk group" (1982, emphasis added). A case can be made that mothers who show little interest in their infants at birth are already displaying a component of abusing behavior. Similarly, children with delayed development in visual/auditory perception can be presumed to be evidencing early signs of a learning disability. In each of these cases, research involving screening for the disorder was based on the incipient symptomatology described (Gray, Cutler, Dean and Kempe, 1979; Silver, Hagin and Beecher, 1978). As the plotting of cumulative risk components approaches maximum prediction accuracy (as the correlation between dispositional factors and the disorder approaches 1.00), a case can be made that what is being observed is not risk but the early manifestations of the disorder itself. It may be argued that these are not instances of primary prevention but early secondary intervention.

Does it really matter? This sort of hair splitting is reminiscent of the puzzle that obsessed medieval scholars involving the number of angels that could dance on the head of a pin. The scholarly quarreling over labels obscures the purpose of interventions with these populations, whether primary or secondary. The point is, after all, to reduce human misery by eliminating, insofar as possible, the conditions that produce dysfunction. The theoretical stalemate signaled by the haggling is instructive. As noted by Kuhn (1970), such stalemates customarily precede a paradigm shift in the scientific community. The common world view shared by scientists permits agreement about which methods to use and which problems to solve. When the methods cease to work and the problems resist solution, a crisis occurs. New methods emerge, along with a new world view and a new set of problems.

The process of replacing an old paradigm with a new one is occurring now in the field of prevention (Rappaport, 1977; Bloom, 1979). The seeds of the new paradigm have been around almost half a century. In 1935, Lewin formulated an equation identifying the critical variables that control behavior: $B = f(PE)$. While it is essentially an unarguable proposition that behavior is a function of the person interacting with the environment, the field of mental health has focused primarily on the person half of the equation. It is only recently that environmental variables have received commensurate attention. The significant relationship between environmental variables and mental illness has been extensively and persuasively documented (Schwab and Schwab, 1978; Insel, 1980). Environmental measures account for more variance in behavior than measures of personality and biographic or demographic variables together.

Community mental health professionals have been slow to recognize the importance of the environment in shaping behavior seemingly because of training, the context in which services are delivered, or the relatively greater access to effecting personal versus environmental changes. In the last decade, however, the search for predisposing factors in the *person* has shifted to a search for precipitating events in the *environment* (Cassel, 1974; Bloom, 1979). This signals a new emphasis on the environmental side of the behavioral equation. High risk situations are seen as responsible for triggering a variety of disorders through the impact of stress. The emergent emphasis on the environment in community mental health has focused almost exclusively on the social environment. As Cassel puts it, "recent investigators have postulated that one of the hitherto overlooked features of the environment of potential importance in disease etiology is the presence of other members of the same species" (1974, p.471). It is notable that the Social Readjustment Rating Scale developed by Holmes and Rahe (1967) reflects this shift. Commonly used as a measure of psychosocial stress, it predicts illness, not as a function of personality or constitutional factors, but as a function of changes occurring in the social environment of the person.

The semantic confusion resulting from the public health definition, and the shift in focus from the person to the environment, has led to a reformulation of the definition of prevention. The old three-level classification has given way to a new triumverate. Whereas the public health definition expanded prevention to cover the universe of community mental health services (prevention, treatment and rehabilitation), the new definition contracts the meaning of prevention to primary prevention and outlines its domain to include disease prevention, health promotion and health protection.

Health promotion embodies an approach of fostering positive behaviors and general health practices primarily through public education and information. Health promotion activities are designed both to encourage individual behavior change and to *improve socioeconomic and physical environments*.

Health protection embodies an approach of fostering general health through public regulatory and control activities, *particularly those related to environmental factors* affecting health, e.g. water purification and chlorination.

Disease prevention encompasses services to prevent the occurrence of specific disorders, using strategies derived from analysis of risk factors for such disorders (Alcohol Drug Abuse and Mental Health Administration Prevention Policy Paper, 1979; 4-6, emphasis added).

The negative connotation of prevention (making something undesirable not happen) has thus been expanded to include positive health prescriptions (making some desirable things happen). This new definition reflects the new consciousness of the significance of environmental variables and suggests preventive strategies for the community mental health field.

THE ROLE OF CONSULTATION AND EDUCATION IN PREVENTION

Prevention is an integral part of the philosophy of the community mental health movement. President John F. Kennedy, in his historic message to Congress dealing with mental health and illness (1963), lent the stature and authority of his office to the goal of preventing mental illness:

> We must seek out the causes of mental illness and of mental retardation and eradicate them. Here, more than in any other area, an ounce of prevention is far more desirable for all concerned. It is far more economical and it is far more likely to be successful. Prevention will require both selected specific programs directed especially at known causes, and the general strengthening of our fundamental community, social welfare, and educational programs which can do much to eliminate or correct the harsh environmental conditions which often are associated with mental retardation and mental illness. (Kennedy, 1963)

The subsequent legislation and regulations launching community mental health centers assigned the prevention task to Consultation and Education (C&E) services:

> Four of the five essential elements of service required in a comprehensive community mental health center focus on new methods of treatment and care. The fifth, consultation and education to community agencies and professionals, is concerned with the prevention of mental illness and the promotion of mental health. (U.S. Department of Health, Education and Welfare, 1966)

The inclusion of prevention as one of the initial five mandated services, coupled with a presidential endorsement, might have been expected to guarantee prevention's fortunes within the new community mental health enterprise; not so. An analysis of community mental health staff hours over the most recent six-year period for which data are available shows that, at their peak, C&E services never exceed 5 percent of the total staff hours available. The parallel with the general health field is striking. Out of every dollar spent for health in the United States, ninety-five cents goes to treatment and five cents to prevention (Surgeon General, 1979). Two further observations make this dismal commitment even sorrier. First, the proportion of C&E hours to total community mental health center hours declined by almost half during this reporting period. Erosion has since given way to rout. While Reaganomics has resulted in the decimation of community mental health center programs in general, C&E programs have suffered proportionately larger cuts than other services (Weiner, Woy, Sharfstein & Bass, 1979). Assigned a "last hired, first fired" status, without the floor funding of grant support or third party reimbursement, the uneasy union of community mental health center treatment and prevention services seems destined to split, or at least to suffer severe estrangement.

Second, it is estimated that not more than half of all C&E activities in community mental health centers can legitimately be labeled as preventive (Perlmutter, 1976). The reasons for the meager allotment of community mental health resources to prevention are documented elsewhere (Snow and Newton, 1976; Swift, 1980). They include the resistance of the medical establishment to prevention, the clinical background and bias of community mental health center administrators, and the lack of training programs for prevention professionals.

How have the limited resources been spent? What types of prevention programs have been implemented by community mental health centers? The common strategies for community mental health prevention programs are reviewed below, and success models are cited. Federal guidelines require the reporting of C&E activities under the categories of case consultation, program consultation, public information and public education, and staff development/continuing education. To facilitate the review these categories are retained.

Consultation

Consultation addresses prevention goals when it is directed toward improving the health of a specified population. When C&E practitioners assist legislative staffs in designing health legislation, or regulatory agencies in formulating policies around such issues as zoning, noise or clean air, the population that benifits is the general public. When the beneficiaries are employees of business and industry, the C&E consultant may be providing the service in the context of an employee assistance program (EAP). Consultations with preventive relevance involve the C&E consultant with representatives of management and labor in developing policies to improve the working conditions and resources of the worker. Consultations with school personnel around formulation of policies for students may also serve prevention goals. According to National Institute of Mental Health (NIMH) categories, these instances are classified as program consultation.

Most consultation activity in community mental health centers, however, is case consultation with a caregiver or significant other about a clinical client. Case consultation is not regarded as a preventive activity since it focuses on the treatment of an individual diagnosed as having emotional, social or behavioral problems. While such consultation could have preventive implications

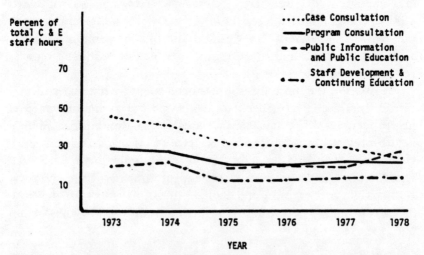

Figure 7-1. Percentage of total C&E staff hours of case consultation, program consultation, public information and public education, and staff development/continuing education from 1973 through 1978 for federally funded community mental health centers. From Ferdinand Hassler, Current national data and trends for consultation and education services. Courtesy of The Staff College, National Institute of Mental Health, May, 1980.

for members of the client's immediate family, and for future students or clients of professionals receiving consultation, its major focus is treatment, not prevention. The largest recipient population for community mental health center case consultation is children, who account for 40 percent of the total hours of delivered services. During the early 1970s, case consultation comprised almost half of all C&E activities in federally funded community mental health centers (Hassler, 1980). As shown in Figure 7-1, this effort *appears* to have declined substantially in subsequent years. I have argued elsewhere (Swift, 1980) that this apparent reduction is an artifact of funding realities and that the same activity is now being reported as a clinical service so as to recover fees.

Program consultation, as noted above, has direct relevance to prevention. It accounts for approximately one-quarter of all C&E activity. Following are the components of program consultation relevant to prevention as defined by the NIMH Contingency Planning Group on Consultation and Education (1974).

— Technical assistance to community commissions or boards charged with planning the direction of mental health related services or activities for the community.
— Consultation to community and governmental organizations for the development of non-mental health programs or facilities having an impact upon the community in areas other than mental health, such as urban renewal, school desegregation, transportation, etc.
— Consultation to national or international agencies on the mental health implications of issues that have an impact on the community (p.4).

Interestingly, this early definition identified another type of consultation that was later lumped into program consultation for reporting purposes:

— *Community Development Consultation* is working in unison with other agencies in the community in planning and devising joint solutions to human service problems. This includes participating in organizational development with agencies whose primary missions are not to render aid to persons under stress but whose operations nevertheless have major implications for the mental health of significant portions of the population (pp. 4-5).

Washtenaw County Community Mental Health Center's work with the Bryant Neighborhoods in Ann Arbor, Michigan (Davidson, 1979; Murphy, Hasenfeld and Rekshan, 1979; Schelkun, 1980) embodies most of the types of program consultation listed above. It is a success model using program consultation in the service of prevention. It began when over 1,000 low income housing units, which came to be known as the Bryant Neighborhoods, were built in a middle-class white neighborhood served by a single school. To cope with the escalating enrollment that resulted, fourteen portable classrooms were moved onto the school grounds. The Parent Teacher Organization, concerned with overcrowding and problems of classroom management that accompanied the tripled enrollment, requested help from the staff of the Washtenaw Center. In response, C&E staff conducted parenting workshops and consulted on volatile school issues.

There were more black, single parent and ADC families among Bryant Neighborhood residents than in the established community. Defaults on mortgages in the low income neighborhood resulted in boarded-up homes and vandalism. The problems expanded from school issues to include the new neighborhood's lack of basic social services and transportation resources. The clash of divergent demographics led — in Ann Arbor as in the rest of the nation in the 1960s — to confrontation and alienation between community groups.

Eventually Bryant Neighborhood residents themselves asked the Washtenaw staff for assistance in coping with the crisis. Center staff began to meet with concerned residents and to involve other community agencies in a search for solutions. An overriding concern of the consultation team was that resident leaders from the Bryant area not be scapegoated by the larger community. To prevent this, consultants focused on defusing the emotional nature of the conflict and advised avoidance of actions that would draw personal attacks. The consultation team focused less on the outcome of the dispute than on the impact the dispute would have on the community in years to come (Davidson, 1979).

What were the specific accomplishments of the Bryant program consultations? Foremost was the organization of a steering committee within Bryant Neighborhoods. Dominated initially by agency representatives, the committee eventually overcame resident apathy and was recognized as the neighborhood's official representative in transactions with the city's political system. Community programs initiated by the committee included a Tot Drop-In Center, a Well Child Clinic, a Boy's Club and a neighborhood newsletter. A critical constant of the preventive effort was the pairing of community mental health center consultants with neighborhood residents for all program tasks, from planning to implementation. One of the C&E consultants completed training as a mortgage counselor. The Department of Housing and Urban Development contributed one of the housing units as a community house. Defaults and vandalism dropped off. The evidence of the integration of Bryant Neighborhoods into the larger community is found in their official participation in the city's political process. A Bryant resident, through election to the city council, was able to insure that his constituency's interests were served. A noxious landfill projected for the neighborhood but opposed by residents to city boards, councils and committees. While the Washpairs were made. Visibility of the neighborhood through city council representation led to the appointment of neighborhood residents to city boards, council and committees. While the Washtenaw staff were not involved in these political developments, their intervention role during the earlier crisis facilitated an empowering of the community to seek and achieve effective solutions to neighborhood problems. Obviously the implications for building community competence were significant.

Today, although the center's commitment of staff has dropped by over 80 percent (from 3.5 to 0.5 full-time staff members), the steering committee, Tot Drop-In Center and Boy's Club are flourishing under community leadership.

This example illustrates both the strengths and weaknesses of the community-resource-development model of program consultation in community mental health. Its effectiveness in building community competency is clear. The youth programs, the park, the daycare center, the paved streets, the informed participation in the political process and the neighborhood newsletter are enough to establish the point. It is more difficult to measure what was *prevented* by the center's efforts. Assuming the center had the resources to monitor employment, defaults, vandalism and episodes of accident and physical and mental illness among the target populations, such figures still would not satisfy the scientific need for either control groups or baseline data or justify conclusions as to the causal efficacy of the intervention. More to the point, few community mental health centers have either the staff resources in research and evaluation or the administrative sanction to conduct sophisticated evaluation of C&E programs. The scant research and evaluation resources that are available are consumed with the task of tracking clinical programs. The dilemma for prevention staff in community mental health centers, then, is that current official commitment of center resources to implement prevention programs is small (estimated at less than 1 percent), and the commitment to evaluate these programs is nonexistent.

Public Information and Public Education

In 1975, centers began reporting the number of hours devoted to public information (PI) and public education (PE) activities. In contrast with the general decline in C&E services across the six years studied, PI and PE services have increased over the years, accounting for almost a third of all C&E services by the late 1970s. Informing people about health options and educating them about the causes of accidents and illness carries the potential of preventing negative outcomes in a variety of target populations.

Definitions of PI and PE in community mental health have evolved over the last twenty years. Public information refers to the unilateral dissemination of health-related information to the public through a variety of channels. While newspapers, radio and television are the major media sources, bulletin boards, billboards, mail campaigns, pamphlets and calendars are sometimes used to reach specific target populations. There is no face-to-face contact between the information purveyor and the public in PI programs. Public education activities, on the other hand, do involve direct contact between CMHC staff and the population targeted. They include workshops, conferences and speeches directed to the general public or some specified subpopulation.

One of the most creative public information campaigns in the field of community mental health is that mounted by Concern Counts, a mental health advocacy organization sponsored by the Kansas City Association for Mental Health (Field, 1981). Operating entirely on monetary and service contributions from the local community, the project has won national recognition for its dramatic and innovative efforts at building community competence. Each year, specific problems in living are selected, and an ad campaign is built around the problem, possible solutions and community resources. In 1980, for example, three campaigns were launched, dealing with stress, growing up, and growing old. Over 35,000 pieces of information on stress were distributed, along with 1,000 "Strike Out Stress" information packets. The local media provided two five-part television series on stress and over forty hours of radio and television coverage for the campaign targeted to the elderly. A peer group communication tool was developed — the "Growing Up Game" — and distributed nationally by the Campfire Girls. More recently, Concern Counts supplied media spots and a television script for a collaborative effort with other mental health agencies in Kansas City following the disaster at the Hyatt Regency Hotel. The goal of the effort was to prevent severe or abnormal grief and shock responses that are often found for the survivors, the families of the victims and the larger community when a disaster of such proportions strikes. Currently, no data are available to evaluate the impact of the program.

The Alternatives project, in Louisville, Kentucky, is a notable exception — evaluation was built into the budget. Sponsored by the River Region Mental Health Mental Retardation Board, Alternatives was an attempt to use the mass media to change public attitudes about common problems and provide positive principles of daily living (Department of HEW, 1975). Intervention was planned in collaboration with an advertising agency. The creative appeal of the messages produced is demonstrated by the awards they attracted: five in local and three in national competitions. The three themes of the campaign were poor interpersonal communication, unmet emotional needs and feelings of alienation and/or depression. While designed for the general public, specific media messages were also adapted to appeal primarily to adolescents or adults. In addition to theme and age, the messages were systematically varied by whether or not the situation depicted was resolved. Half showed the character(s) resolving the problem and half showed the situation as unresolved.

In all, the sixty-week media blitz consisted of sixteen different ads in seventeen newspapers, thirty radio spots from thirty to sixty seconds each aired on eighteen stations (four spots a day were scheduled to be run on each station), twenty-one television spots to be broadcast on five local stations at the rate of ten messages each week, 2,000 cards placed inside buses, a slide presentation for civic groups, and 1,500 reprints of ads distributed to churches, industry and schools. The project budgeted almost $14,000 to evaluate the impact of the prevention messages (the goals and budget related to the clinical program are not reported here).

The results demonstrate a number of lessons for those who would use the media in health campaigns. Through surveys it was found that 40 percent of the subjects recalled one or more of the mental health messages. Television was more powerful than radio in having an impact on audiences. While 67 percent of persons surveyed recalled viewing one or more messages on television, only 7 percent of these reported hearing the radio messages. In total, 22 percent reported exposure from both media.

Demographic analysis revealed that younger people and the more affluent and better educated segments of the audience surveyed recalled significantly more of the messages. One of the more useful findings for future media campaigns is the messages featuring unresolved endings were recalled significantly more often than those depicting resolutions – the Zeigarnik Effect is alive and well in community mental health.

The results on the critical issue of attitude change are mixed. Significant shifts in attitude were demonstrated on almost half of the mental health survey items (18 out of 39). A disconcerting result, however, was that a third of these changes were in the wrong direction. Unfortunately, the survey items were not pretested. Therefore, post hoc conclusions about the ambiguity of certain items cannot be proven. The report concludes that, on balance, media intervention brought about positive attitude change in the audience.

A major barrier to the widespread implementation of prevention programs has been the difficulty in reaching target populations. As the Alternatives project demonstrated, one of the most effective means of reaching the general population is through the medium of television. Children in this country watch an average of three to four hours of television daily (Comstock, 1977). By the age of eighteen, today's children will have spent more time watching television than hours in the classroom (Liebert, Neale & Davidson, 1973). In the average American household, the set is on seven hours a day (Comstock, Chaffee, Katzman & McCombs, 1978).

In addition to providing entertainment, television is both a social support and an educator. As a social support it is a baby-sitter, a companion for the lonely, and a catalyst for social interaction. As an educational tool it teaches from *A* to *Z* from the alphabet to highly technical scientific material. The parameters of learning through television have only been marginally explored to date. The five volumes of technical reports to the Surgeon General's Scientific Advisory Committee on Television and Social Behavior (1972) document the role of television in teaching aggressive behaviors to children (Liebert & Baron, 1973; McCarthy, Langner, Gerston, Eisenberg & Orzeck, 1975; Meyer, 1973). While television's capacity to teach violence has been experimentally explored and confirmed, less attention has been given to an examination of the medium's capacity to teach prosocial behaviors, even though available research indicates that learning of prosocial behavior does take place (Harvey, Sprafkin & Rubenstein, 1979; Liebert & Poulos, 1975; Liebert, Sprafkin & Poulos, 1974; Liebert, Sprafkin & Poulos, 1974; Sprafkin & Rubenstein, 1979). The recommendations for future research from the Summary Report to the Surgeon General (1972, p.11) cite the influence of the home environment and the modeling and imitation of prosocial behavior as two priority subjects. The community mental health field in general has ignored the potential television holds for prevention programming, although the subject is currently under review (Sprafkin, Swift & Hess, in press).

The revolution in media resources over the past decade has put at our fingertips the potential for influencing the behavior of vast numbers of persons. Industries with commercial projects have been quick to use market research to identify audiences and direct sales promotions. The cost of one minute of prime time television advertising testifies to the success of these efforts. A brief review of recent findings in television research conveys the potential of this medium for affecting attitudes and behavior. Children viewing television in pairs are more likely to imitate filmed aggressive behavior than children viewing alone (Drabman & Thomas, 1977). Over 70 percent of the content of major network news programs presents some form of helplessness on the part of the central figure (Levine, 1977), raising the question of whether these programs are teaching "learned helplessness" (reference Seligman, 1975). Heavy television viewers are more likely than light viewers to report feelings of general mistrust, caution, and insecurity (Gerbner & Gross, 1976). Adolescents rate viewing television with their parents as more productive to social learning than viewing with siblings, friends or alone (Chaffee & Tims, 1976).

The major primary prevention television study aimed at a mass audience and targeted to changing behaviors having an impact on health is the Stanford study (Maccoby & Farquhar, 1975, 1976). While this study is directed to reducing heart disease — on the surface a health rather than mental health problem — it targets behavior change, rather than medical intervention, as the method for accomplishing reduction. Attempts to change behaviors associated with diet, weight loss, exercise and smoking cessation put the intervention squarely in mental health territory. Researchers at Stanford University conducted a study using the mass media and individual instruction to reduce susceptibility to heart disease. Three California towns were selected for participation: Gilroy, Watsonville and Tracy. Tracy was outside the mass media orbit of the other two towns. The behaviors targeted for change were smoking, diet, and exercise. Surveys of persons aged thirty-five to thirty-nine were conducted in samples drawn from each city to assess attitudes and determine baseline measures of the target behaviors. Medical examinations provided assessment of subjects on the Cornfield Scale of risk for heart disease. Subjects in Watsonville scoring in the highest 20 percent of this scale were selected for a special program of intensive instruction.

The media campaign, which covered Watsonville and Gilroy only, included:

television — forty spot announcements

radio — spot announcements and mini-dramas

newspaper — doctor's column, diet columns

direct mail — cookbook, basic information booklet, health calendar

other — billboards, business cards

Results indicate that target behaviors and attitudes in the two towns receiving the mass media programs changed in the predicted direction more than those in the control town. In addition, those high risk subjects who received media intervention *plus* special instruction showed greater change after the first year of the intervention than those who received media messages alone. After the second year, however, the media-alone group made comparable gains to the media-plus instruction group in all areas except smoking reduction.

Behavioral changes included reductions in smoking and egg consumption. Attitude changes were also noted relating to diet and injury to health caused by smoking. No changes were observed in physical exercise or weight loss. The medical indicators of the high risk group receiving intensive instruction showed substantial improvement on the Cornfield Scale. While initial evaluation showed the clear superiority of the combination of intensive instruction and mass media (Watsonville) over mass media alone (Gilroy), subsequent evaluation showed the two towns to be essentially equivalent.

These findings demonstrate what major corporations have known all along, but what health professionals are just beginning to discover: bombarding viewers with a simple message gets results. It sells cereal, toothpaste and cars. The Stanford study demonstrates that it can also sell health. The expansion of cable television services across the country, coupled with the requirements of most communities that citizen groups be permitted access to programming, makes television an attractive option for implementing prevention programs. The lack of knowledge and training of community mental health center professionals in the technology of television productions has, so far, limited such programs. Despite such limitations, dozens of community mental health centers are currently experimenting with a variety of programs directed at changing public attitudes, promoting health and preventing disease.[1]

Media health campaigns, in general, have not been as successful as had been hoped. Reasons for the lack of success include (1) failure to pretest materials (Kotler & Zaltman, 1971); (2) failure to segment the audience demographically and tailor the appeal to the targeted segments (Mendelsohn, 1973); (3) focusing too narrowly on the long-range goal of behavior change without attention to the medium-range goal of attitude change (Mendelsohn, 1973); (4) failure to specify actions or procedures by which members of the audience can change their habits or life-styles (Weibe, 1951); and (5) unrealistic expectations about the proportion of the audience that can be influenced to change. Marketers of a commercial media campaign may count it as a success if 1 or 2 percent of the audience buys the product; considering the millions exposed, this may translate into hundreds of thousands of dollars (Weibe, 1951). It is unlikely that prevention professionals would be satisfied with such a minimal impact.

Public Education

Public education services usually involve the practitioner and the recipient in face-to-face contact. The purpose of mental health education is to build coping skills as a result of competent training and to prepare normal or at-risk groups to deal more effectively with stress and predictable life crises (such as birth, marriage, parenting and death). Is early intervention legitimately classified as prevention? Criticism levelled at many PE programs echoes the objections raised about prevention programs with r–igh risk populations. It is true that many of the educational offerings of community mental health centers are directed toward those lacking in targeted skills. Parenting classes for abusing parents, assertiveness training for passive people, and stress management for the anxious serve treatment rather than prevention goals. However, the issue is not as simple as it seems. These same classes, when offered to the

---

[1] Paul Kradel, C&E Director with the Appalachian Mental Health Center in Elkins, West Virginia, is an individual who is able to provide guidelines and specific instructions for the use of the media for community education.

general public, may include participants from both high and low risk populations. When multiple risk are involved, the proportion of the population that meets the risk criteria may expand to approach the general population census.

An increasingly popular prevention program in community mental health centers consists of early intervention and infant stimulation activities for pregnant women and mothers of newborn babies who are considered to be at-risk for the development of a range of negative outcomes — child abuse, retardation, developmental delay, school behavior problems, etc. For many of these programs, pregnant women are considered to be at-risk if the woman has any one of a variety of medical conditions, e.g. hypertension, cardiovascular or pulmonary disorders; is under sixteen years of age or is middle aged (over 40); is unwed, malnourished, smokes, or is addicted to drugs or alcohol; has suffered trauma during pregnancy, or has a history of reproductive failures, difficult labor or pre- or postterm delivery. In one such program, currently being implemented in Columbus, Ohio, some 95 percent of the women served by the local health center meet the risk criteria.

Whatever the nuances of classification, early intervention and infant stimulation programs in general *are* demonstrating positive results. The Optimum Growth Project, sponsored by the South County Mental Health Center in Delray Beach, Florida, won the first Lela Rowland Prevention Award presented by the Mental Health Association (South County Mental Health Center, Inc., 1980). Using paraprofessional staff as the primary service deliverers, home visits are made to pregnant women, mothers and children and continue through the infant's first year, followed by biweekly visits through the age of three and follow-up contacts as needed until the child attains six years of age. The visits consist of parenting activity, modeled by the worker for the mother, across some 200 tasks involving infant stimulation. The mental health worker functions as a support to the family by providing parenting education and facilitating referrals to other social service agencies further to meet the families' needs. Voluntary parent groups are also a part of the program.

An evaluation conducted during the third year of the six-year program showed that the mothers in the test group (those receiving the home visits) improved significantly when compared to control group mothers in caring for their children's physical needs and interacting with their children, e.g. hugging, eye contact. In addition, 25 percent of the test mothers had returned to work. A most striking finding is that "Less than one percent of test group mothers had been reported for child abuse and neglect as compared 7.7 percent of comparison group mothers" (p.7). Preliminary results for the children in the study show that 2.1 percent of the test children scored below 100 on the Mental and Motor Section of the Bayley Scales of Infant Development, compared with 15.6 percent of the control children. Attempts to relate the results to demographic factors through multiple regression analysis demonstrated significant differences between Bayley scores of children of teenage mothers and other children. These impressive results provide evidence that the use of home visits, in combination with parenting groups, is an effective format for delivering mental health education services.

Staff Development/Continuing Education

A final category of C&E services tracked by NIMH is labeled "staff development/continuing education" services and involves the training of caregivers and professionals in agencies other than the community mental health center delivering the service. This activity has consistently accounted for approximately one-fifth of all community mental health center C&E services. Almost 40 percent of such training is targeted at schools and other agencies dealing with children. Training teachers to assist children in learning problem-solving skills or in managing their classrooms more effectively has obvious implications for prevention.

One of the most widely replicated models of staff development/caregiver training is that developed by Myrna Shure and George Spivack and is designed to improve children's interpersonal cognitive problem-solving skills (ICPS) (Shure & Spivack, 1972, 1974; Spivack & Shure, 1974). Nursery, elementary and secondary school teachers are taught how to present the basic problem-solving curriculum, which is designed to be integrated into the regular classroom routine. The curriculum assists children in learning a broad repertoire of problem-solving techniques ranging from simple listening and language skills to concepts of logic (if-then, either-or, both-and), multiple attributes and labeling emotions. A daily lesson script of games, scheduled to last approximately twenty minutes, aids teachers in presenting the material. The *Preschool Interpersonal Problem Solving Scale* (PIPS) (Shure & Spivack, 1974) serves as a pretest and posttest measure of the success of the intervention. An early evaluation of the program found that children who received training in their classrooms were able to generate significantly more solutions on the PIPS than children who did not receive training (Shure & Spivack, 1975). A further measure of program effectiveness, which has short-term prevention implications, is found in teacher reports of behavioral change on the part of nursery school children receiving the ICPS training. Significantly fewer children were judged by teachers to be impulsive or inhibited during their kindergarten year. While the ultimate target population for intervention is the children themselves, training teachers to present the program multiplies the program's positive effects across entire educational systems.

This "multiplier" effect is the rationale behind the strategy of staff development or caregiver training. A variety of community mental health center programs have been developed to train persons whose responsibilities place them in direct contact with the public, including clergy, police, social service case workers, hair dressers and bartenders. The social problems targeted for prevention range from domestic problems such as divorce, spouse and child abuse to problems of addiction, depression and suicide.

WHAT LIES AHEAD?

This brief sampling of prevention activity in the community mental health field leads logically to an attempt to assess the direction and commitment of the field to ongoing prevention activities. At a time when the future of the entire community mental health movement is in question, due to the rescinding of the Mental Health Systems Act and the shift to a reduced funding of block grants, it is difficult to make predictions. However, four trends seem clear. These include (1) a transfer of the control of prevention programs from the federal government to the states; (2) a reduction of C&E programs — and thus prevention — in community mental health centers; (3) a growing commitment to prevention programs in health and human service agencies *outside of* community mental health centers; and (4) an increasing rapprochément between the fields of health and mental health in the implementation of prevention programs.

Even before the Reagan administration's transfer of funding and control of community mental health programs from the federal to the state level, the process had already begun. The Mental Health Systems Act, in its Title II, established prevention authorities within state governments and provided funds for staff, research and training to develop prevention expertise at the local level. There are both advantages and disadvantages to this shift of authority to the state. One of the disadvantages is states' historical responsibility to maintain state hospitals for the mentally ill. This commitment, in most states, has involved the state mental health bureaucracy in funding beds in antiquated institutions, thus perpetuating a mental health industry that may or may not reflect the needs of the people served. The states' traditional commitment to hospitalizing the mentally ill puts the community mental health movement and the state on a collision course with regard to the expenditure of state mental health dollars. This was not a problem in the "boom" years, when the "Godfather," as Saul Cooper (1981) referred to the federal government, took care of the community mental health centers with direct largesse. Now, however, with the "Godfather" in retirement, state mental health authorities and community mental health centers are left to divide the greatly reduced mental health dollars between them. The process of arriving at consensus promises to be a painful one.

Another disadvantage of placing control of community mental health programs at the state level is the inevitable exacerbation of local political pressures that could result. Urban and rural areas will likely be pitted against each other in an effort to win a share of diminished mental health dollars.

The ostensible advantage of the shift of authority from the federal to the state level is at the ideological heart of the *community* mental health movement: local programs should reflect local priorities. By placing decision-making power at the local level, the argument goes, community mental health programs are more likely to represent the needs of the local community. The problem with this argument is the existing inequity in the distribution of services, which the Mental Health Systems Act sought to redress. In the field of community mental health, underserved and unserved populations exist throughout the country. These include minorities, children, the elderly, the chronically mentally disabled and the poor. Left to their own resources, without the incentives of grants, local communities may tend to slight these populations in mental health as in other social services. While local control can be regarded as an opportunity for communities to assert and enforce their won priorities, the danger remains that a large part of the population in need of mental health services will be overlooked.

A second trend is the reduction of community mental health center prevention resources. As noted earlier, C&E — and thus prevention — services are currently suffering a proportionately larger share of budget cuts than clinical services. In many cases, C&E units are being eliminated and the staff either laid off or drafted into clinical service. This raises the question as to whether the community mental health movement can sustain the current delivery model for prevention, i.e. out of community mental health centers, or whether these services will be delivered primarily through other agencies in the future. Perlmutter (1974), during the largesse of the "Godfather" era, predicted that prevention staff would eventually be forced to seek professional homes outside of treatment agencies, just as prevention and treatment are generally separated in the field of physical and medical health. Hospitals minister to the ill and health centers to the well — through programs of innoculations, screening, family planning and well baby/child clinics. Perlmutter sees prevention and treatment as incompatible within the same agency for ideological, organizational and professional reasons. Ignoring the differing philosophies of treatment and prevention, the bottom line remains. Sick people pay to get well, or arrange to have their treatment paid through insurance. Few well people will pay community mental health centers to stay that way. The current dogma in these years of retrenchment is that social service programs that do not pay for themselves are doomed to extinction in today's economy.

At the same time that community mental health centers are reducing their commitment to prevention, the concept is gaining respect in health and medicine (Surgeon General, 1979), labor and industry (ADAMHA, 1981), and the proliferation of regulatory agencies charged with preventing exposure to toxic substances in the environment — both natural and manufactured. Munoz (1976) notes that, in fact, "most well-designed prevention work has not come from mental health centers" (p.11). That the public refuses to pay for prevention is belied by the success of preventive phenomena such as health spas, books on such topics as diet, stress, assertiveness and exercise, and the millions of dollars spent on vitamins each year. While most of these innovations are dedicated to preventing physical illness, all require changes in behavior and lifestyle on the part of their adherents.

The final trend noted is the decline of the traditional dichotomy between health and mental health. This is seen in the holistic health movement, the development of scholarly journals dealing with stress, the emergence of health education as a physical strategy, and the emphasis on linkages between health and mental health systems. Multiple systems point to the convergence of the fields of health and mental health in human service delivery.

What do these trends mean for community mental health center prevention services? First, unless prevention professionals in these centers practice aggressive "outreach" to link with their counterparts in other human service agencies, particularly health agencies, prevention activities in community mental health centers will be reduced or become nonexistent over the next decade. Second, to survive, prevention programs in community mental health centers will need to be marketed to their communities more effectively than in the past. This process will involve selling decision makers as well as the general public on the desirability of prevention programs. Third, the change from the expansion mode of the past to the current mode of contraction also means it is unlikely that the field of community mental health will make significant contributions to the new paradigm being articulated among prevention theorists today. The emphasis on precipitating factors in situations that lead to disorder signals attempts to control environmental conditions. System change in an increasingly conservative political and economic climate will be an option available to few community mental health centers. Therefore, the preventive interventions characteristic of CMHCs in the 1980s will be focused on changing individuals rather than environments. Fourth, community mental health centers that are able to maintain a prevention function will likely do so through fewer staff-intensive prevention strategies, such as public information and public education.

In summary, economic realities dictate a restriction of preventive strategies for community mental health centers over the short term. The challenge for the community mental health movement lies, ultimately, in its capacity to deliver on its early promise to prevent mental illness. Here the crystal ball is clouded. The outcome is unknown. Nevertheless, it is some comfort to reflect that the concept of prevention exhibits the tenacity, the guile and the simple but powerful wisdom embodied in folktales — which, as every child knows, long outlive their narrators.

REFERENCES

1. ADAMHA. Policy Paper on Prevention. Office of the Administrator, Office of Program Planning and Coordination, Division of Prevention, 1979, 4-6.
2. ———. Conference on prevention at the worksite. Washington, D.C., June 16 and 17, 1981.
3. Anthony, J. E. Preventive measures for children and adolescents at high risk for psychosis. In George Albee & Justin Joffee (Eds.), *Primary prevention of psychopathology, I: The Issues.* The University Press of New England, 1977, 164-174.
4. Bell, R., & Pearl, D. Psychosocial change in risk groups: implications for early identification. *Journal of Prevention in Human Services,* in press.
5. Bloom, B. Prevention of mental disorders: Recent advances in theory and practice. *Community Mental Health Journal,* 1979, *13*(3) 179-191.
6. Cassel, J. Psychosocial processes and "stress": Theoretical formulation. *Journal of Health Services,* 1974, 4 (3) 471-481.
7. Chaffee, S. H., & Tims, A. R. Interpersonal factors in adolescent television use. *The Journal of Social Issues,* 1976, *32*(4), 98-115.

8. Comstock, G., Chaffee, S., Katzman, N., McCombs, M. & Roberts, D. *Television and human behavior.* New York: Columbia University Press, 1978.

9. Cooper, S. Changing consultation and education: New ground rules. Address presented at the National Council of Community Mental Health Centers Region I Annual Conference, Hartford, Connecticut, November 11, 1981.

10. Cowen, E. The wooing of primary prevention. *American Journal of Community Psychology,* 1980, *8*(3), 253-284.

11. Davidson, J. *Political partnerships: Neighborhood residents and their council members.* Beverly Hills, Cal.: Sage Publications, 1979.

12. Drabman, R., & Thomas, M. Children's imitation of aggressive and prosocial behavior when viewing alone and in pairs. *Journal of Communication,* 1977, *27*(3), 199-205.

13. Field, J. Personal communication, September 14, 1981.

14. Gerbner, G. & Gross, L. Living with television: The violence profile. *Journal of communication,* 1976, *26*(2), 173-199.

15. Gray, J., Cutler, C., Dean, J., & Kempe, C. Prediction and prevention of child abuse. *Seminars in Perinatology,* 1979, *3,* 85-90.

16. Harvey, S., Sprafkin, J., & Rubinstein, E. Prime time television: A profile of aggressive and prosocial behaviors. *Journal of Broadcasting,* 1979, *23*(2), 179-189.

17. Hassler, F. Current national data and trends for consultation and education services. The Staff College, National Institute of Mental Health, May, 1980.

18. Holmes, R., & Rahe, R. The social adjustment rating scale. *Journal of Psychosomatic Research,* 1967, *11,* 213-218.

19. Insel, P. M. *Environmental variables and the prevention of mental illness.* New York: Lexington Books, 1980.

20. Kennedy, J. Message to Congress from the President of the United States relative to mental health and mental retardation. February 5, 1963.

21. Kessler, M., & Albee, G.W. Primary Prevention. *Annual Review of Psychology,* 1975, *26,* 557-591.

22. Kotler, P., & Zaltman, G. Social marketing: An approach to planned social change. *Journal of Marketing,* 1971, *35,* 3-12.

23. Kradel, P. Use of media outlets for community education. Mimeo. 1980.

24. Kuhn, T.S. *The structure of scientific revolutions* (2nd ed.) Chicago: University of Chicago Press, 1970.

25. Levine G. "Learned helplessness" and the evening news. *Journal of Communication,* 1977, *27*(4), 100-105.

26. Lewin, Kurt. *A dynamic theory of personality.* New York: McGraw Hill, 1935.

27. Liebert, R. M., Neale, J.M., & Davidson, E.S. *The early window: Effects of television on children and youth.* Elmsford, New York: Pergammon Press, 1973.

28. Liebert, R.M., & Poulos, R.W. Television and personality development: The socializing effects of an entertainment medium. In A. Davids (Ed.), *Child personality and psychopathology* (Vol. 2). New York: Wiley, 1975.

29. Liebert, R.M., Sprafkin, J.N., & Poulos, R.W. In William S. Hale (Ed.), *20th Annual Conference/1974 Proceedings.* Advertising Research Foundation, 1975, 54-57.

30. Maccoby, N., & Farquhar, J. Communication for health: Unselling heart disease. *Journal of Communication,* 1975, *25*(3), 115-126.

31. ———. Bringing the California health report up to date. *Journal of Communication,* 1976, *26*(1), 56-57.

32. McCarthy, E.D., Langner, T. S., Gersten, J. C., Eisenberg, J. G., & Orzeck, L. Violence and behavior disorders. *Journal of Communication,* 1975, *25*(4), 71-75.

33. Mendelsohn, H. Some reasons why information campaigns can succeed. *Public Opinion Quarterly,* 1973, *37*(1), 50-60.

34. Munoz, R. The primary prevention of psychological problems. *Community Health Review,* 1976, *1*(6), 1-14.

35. Murphy, M., Hasenfeld, H., & Rekshan, L. Lend lease consultation. Presentation made at the annual meeting of the National Council of Community Mental Health Centers, San Francisco, February, 1980.

36. NIMH Contingency Planning Group on Consultation and Education. Report. 1974.

37. Perlmutter, F. D. Prevention and treatment: A strategy for survival. *Community Mental Health Journal,* 1974, *10,* 276-281.

38. ———. An instrument for differentiating in prevention — primary, secondary and tertiary. *American Journal of Orthopsychiatry,* 1976, *46,* 533-541.

39. Rappaport, Julian. *Community psychology: Values, research and action.* New York: Holt, Rinehart & Winston, 1977.

40. Schelkun, R. Personal communication, February 9, 1980.

41. Schwab, J., & Schwab, M. *Sociocultural roots of mental illness: An epidemiological survey.* New York: Plenum, 1978.

42. Shure, M.B., & Spivack, G. *Preschool Interpersonal Problem-Solving (PIPS) Test: Manual.* Philadelphia: Department of Mental Health Sciences, Hahnemann Medical College and Hospitals, 1974.

43. Shure, M.B., Spivack, G., & Gordon, R. Problem-solving thinking: A preventive mental health program for preschool children. *Reading World*, 1972, *11*, 259-273.

44. Seligman, M.P. Depression and learned helplessness. In D. Rosehan & P. London (Eds.), *Theory and research in abnormal psychology* (2nd ed.). New York: Holt, Rinehart & Winston, 1975.

45. Silver, A.A., Hagin, R.A., & Beecher, R. Scanning: Diagnosis and intervention in prevention of reading disability. Part I, Search: The scanning measures. *Journal of Learning Disabilities*, 1978, *11*, 434-445.

46. Snow, D.L., & Newton, P.M. Task, social structure and social process in the community mental health center movement. *American Psychologist*, 1976, *31*, 582-594.

47. South County Mental Health Center. A nomination of the Lela Rowland prevention award 1980: The Optimum Growth project, July, 1980.

48. Spivack, G., & Shure, M.B. *Social adjustment of young children: A cognitive approach to solving real-life problems.* San Francisco: Jossey-Bass, 1974.

49. Sprafkin, J.N., & Rubinstein, E. A field correlation study of children's television viewing habits and prosocial behavior. *Journal of Broadcasting*, 1979.

50. Sprafkin, J., Swift, C., & Hess, R. (Eds). *Rx television: Enhancing the preventive impact of T. V.* New York: Haworth Press, in press.

51. Surgeon General's Report on Health Promotion and Disease Prevention. *Healthy people* (DHEW (PHS) Publication No. 79-55701). Washington, D.C.: U.S. Government Printing Office, 1979.

52. Surgeon General's Scientific Advisory Committee on Television and Social Behavior. *Television and growing up: The impact of televised violence* (summary report). Washington, D.C.: U.S. Government Printing Office, 1972.

53. Swift, C. Primary prevention: Policy and practice. In Richard Price, Richard Ketterer, Barbara Bader, & John Monahan (Eds.), *Prevention in mental health*. Beverly Hills, Cal.: Sage Publications, 1980.

54. United States Department of Health, Education and Welfare. *Essential services of the community mental health center: Consultation and education.* Pamphlet. Washington, D.C.: U.S. Government Printing Office, 1966.

55. ———. *Communicating: How? A manual for mental health educators* (DHEW Publication No. (ADM) 76-290). Washington, D.C.: U.S Government Printing Office, 1975.

56. Vance, E.T. A typology of risks and the disabilities of low status. In George Albee & Justin Joffee (Eds.), *Primary prevention of psychopathology: The issues* (Vol. I). The University Press of New England, 1977, 207-237.

57. Weibe, G. Merchandising commodities and citizenship on television. *Public Opinion Quarterly*, 1951-1952, *Winter*, 679-691.

58. Weiner, J., Woy, R., Sharfstein, S., & Bass, R. Community mental health centers and the "seed money" concept: Effects of terminating federal funds. *Community Mental Health Journal*, 1979, *15*, 129-138.

Chapter 8

PROSPECTS FOR THE FUTURE

DAVID R. RITTER

THIS book has offered a historical perspective, a description of present day practices and a look toward the future prospects of mental health consultation, education and prevention. Each of the contributing authors has explored a different facet of the entity we call C&E. Together, the chapters reflect the pooled knowledge of experienced C&E practitioners and offer an in-depth look at organizational structures, staff development needs, financing strategies, consultation approaches, educational methodologies and preventive programming. Overall, it serves as a representation of the state of the art of Consultation and Education services as they exist today, not in theory, but in reality.

Consultation and Education is one of the most fledgling of mental health services. It has yet to develop a rich history of tradition, and those individuals who could be considered to be mentors in C&E are few. Yet, C&E represents a potential that traditional mental health services cannot begin to match. It is the potential embodied in prevention, but it is a potential that can only be realized if C&E's growth and development are sustained. The onus for this growth is on each of us as C&E practitioners, and it is our task to confront and overcome the challenges that C&E faces.

THE CHALLENGE OF INTEGRATION

It has been said by some that C&E is still engaged in a struggle for identity and that it has yet to define itself. I strongly disagree with such a statement and feel that it does little but continue to perpetuate a myth that pales in the face of reality. It may be true that C&E services have yet to attain the recognition they deserve as an integral rather than fringe service of a mental health center. However, it is inappropriate to interpret this peripheral status as a lack of identity on the part of C&E. I would suggest that C&E possesses the greatest identity of all mental health services. It is C&E's public information and educational programs that are the main factor in promoting an awareness of mental health within the community, and it is the consultation service that receives the greatest recognition on the part of the educational systems. Of all mental health staff, it is the C&E practitioners alone who represent themselves through the use of their functional titles (consultant or educator) rather than their training discipline. Only two CMHC programs, C&E and Inpatient, are commonly referred to as *units* rather than services, once again reflecting a sense of cohesion felt by C&E staff. On a national or regional level, it is C&E alone that conducts an annual conference devoted to its specialty. Clearly, C&E staff *do* possess a strong identity. Although some may view C&E as being outside of the mainstream of mental health services, C&E itself surely knows *who* it is and *what* it needs to do. The crisis is not one of identity but one of acceptance of C&E on the part of those who fail to realize its value or potential.

The factors that provide C&E with a strong sense of identity can also promote its isolation, and I believe it is for this reason that a meaningful integration of C&E and clinical services has never occurred within community mental health. There are those C&E practitioners who would take issue with this statement, arguing that C&E's isolation is a function of a lack of understanding and acceptance on the part of clinicians. To some degree this argument has merit. Yet, one cannot overlook the role that C&E has played in keeping itself apart from mainstream mental health services and the threat to C&E's distinct identity that accompanies a greater integration of C&E and clinical services. It is this conflict of identity versus integration that may well be the foremost issue confronting C&E.

With the advent of the New Federalism, reductions in social programs and transition from categorical to block grant funding make it imperative that C&E begin to align itself with other services of the mental health center. The issue is one of survival, and survival must supersede all other concerns. This does not mean that C&E must subjugate itself to clinical services that it must necessarily lose its own sense of identity. It does mean that C&E will need to discard many of the visible trappings of its differentness in favor of a public image of commonality and coordination. C&E is more than capable of meeting the challenge. After all, there is not another CMHC service that has demonstrated a greater capacity for developing linkages and networks among service providers. It is only that such linkages are intra-agency instead of inter-agency.

THE CHALLENGE OF CREDIBILITY

As C&E redirects some of its energy internally, that is toward the development of within-agency linkages, it may also face the question of the credibility of its services. Consultation, education and prevention are somewhat alien to clinicians, and the value of these services may come into question because they are not fully appreciated. C&E's expertise in education may need to be brought to bear in introducing these concepts to clinicians, furthering their understanding and gradually involving them in C&E practices.

The promotion of awareness and understanding of C&E services on the part of non-C&E staff is but a first step along the road to attaining service credibility. C&E must also demonstrate the benefit of its services, benefit being defined as a meaningful level of consumer demand for C&E services, the impact of consultation or education upon community systems, and the cost-effectiveness of preventive intervention. Thus, program evaluation becomes an essential ingredient for the C&E program of the 1980s.

Initially, C&E would do well to review its service delivery system of recent years for the purpose of documenting consumer demand for and satisfaction with services. This information should be made known to the center's executive director and governing board. C&E's educational programs offer an excellent source of consumer information. For example, data might be compiled on the amount of educational programs offered over the past few years, the number of individuals from the community who attended these seminars or courses and levels of participant satisfaction. Should the participant group have included individuals who are considered to be prominent in the community, such as local or state legislators, heads of other community caregiving systems, or persons who are influential simply because of their community role or status, then a secondary value may be accruing from C&E services, that being the promotion of the public image of the community mental health center. The importance of positive public relations is a point that is well taken by CMHC executive directors, who, themselves, carry ongoing concerns regarding how positively or poorly the CMHC is viewed by the community. Certainly, consumer participant and satisfaction information is but one source of information on the benefit of C&E services, and if harder data on the impact or outcome of C&E services can be compiled, so much the better.

Beyond the perceived or documented value of C&E services, and any accompanying "image" benefits that derive to the CMHC, looms the question of cost-effectiveness. The primary focus of CMHCs during the 1970s was monitoring growth as new services were being developed and implemented constantly in response to community requests and with the support and ready accessibility of state and federal monies. Today, and for the foreseeable future, the major administrative concerns of CMHCs are fiscal with terms such as "cut-back management," "profit-minded management" and "maximizing productivity" being the phraseology of the times. With the flow of federal and state dollars now receding to a trickle, CMHCs are forced to look toward local sources of financial support for the continuation of community services. This situation places C&E at a decided disadvantage when competing for funds with clinical services, given C&E's historical tendency of ignoring the need to generate dollars. The continued viability of C&E as a community mental health center service will depend on the degree to which C&E is able to generate its own financial support and move toward fiscal self-sufficiency. Those C&E programs who are unable or unwilling to address this issue seriously will simply go out of existence.

THE CHALLENGE OF SERVICES

Regardless of how well C&E promotes an awareness of its services, documents its effectiveness and generates its own financial support, I believe it is inevitable that C&E programs will decrease in size. They will face a consolidation of services. Some reductions will occur as natural extensions of a matching of services to the actual level of consumer demand for them and a conscious transition from free to fee for services. C&E practitioners who hold to the adage of "bigger is better" will face a significant value conflict in the coming years as they confront the necessity of reducing both services and staff. C&E, as with other CMHC services, must begin to differentiate between essential services and those which are less crucial, even though they may have proven to be beneficial. The choices will not be easy ones. Additionally, decisions will need to be made on C&E staffing patterns, and it is likely that the relative value of professional versus paraprofessional and specialist versus generalist staff will again see much discussion. C&E staffing patterns will more than ever need to reflect the nature of C&E service priorities. Although prediction is a tenous practice, it seems probable that C&E staff possessing a more generalized expertise and a capacity for multiple service roles will survive their more specialized or service-limited counterparts. I would also anticipate the relative importance of the management skills of C&E directors and coordinators will also see change. Expertise is fiscal and human resource management will take precedence over skills related to the development of programs. In effect, the coordination of services will play a secondary role to the *management* of resources. The maximization of productive staff time in the delivery of *direct* consultation, education or prevention services will be a significant factor in optimally using scarce resources.

CRISIS OR OPPORTUNITY?

It goes without saying that the 1980s have brought with them a number of major challenges, even crises, for community mental health. These crises will have an impact upon community mental health services to varying degrees with services to the chronic mentally disabled population likely to be affected the least and consultation and education services perhaps affected the most. It is, therefore, incumbent for C&E to act on its own behalf — and to act now! Indeed, consultation, education and prevention services face challenges in the coming years, but with such challenge comes the opportunity for vitality and renewal. Whether C&E grasps the opportunity or succumbs to the crises is the remaining question.

NAME INDEX

A

Abidin, R., 122, 141
Adams, G., 20, 44
Adelson, D., 24, 42
Ahmed, P., 16, 45
Albee, G., 25, 37, 40, 42, 44, 171, 196
Andrulis, D., 9, 45
Anthony, J., 171, 195

B

Bader, B., 10, 13, 18, 29, 30, 34, 35, 38, 41, 45
Baizerman, N., 42
Bass, R., 42, 177, 199
Beck, K., 161, 169
Beecher, R., 173, 198
Bell, R., 173, 195
Berlin, I., 15, 42
Biller, H., 32, 43
Blackburn, J., 137, 141
Blackford, V., 42
Bloom, B., 25, 42, 174, 195
Bransford, D., 160, 169
Brock, G., 38, 43
Brown, D., 137, 141
Brown, R., 139, 141

C

Campbell, D., 152, 169
Caplan, G., 14, 15, 17, 42, 127, 132, 133, 141
Caplan, R., 17, 41
Carr, R., 160, 169
Cassel, J., 174, 175, 195
Chaffee, S., 185, 186, 195, 196
Chandler, L., 123, 139, 141
Cherness, C., 16, 20, 42

Chinskey, J., 32, 45
Cline, D., 160, 169
Cohen, L., 126, 141
Collins, A., 17, 43
Comstock, G., 185, 196
Cooper, J., 160, 169
Cooper, S., 15, 19, 44, 192, 196
Cowen, E., 38, 43, 172, 196
Cumming, E., 22, 43
Cumming, J., 22, 43
Cutler, C., 173, 196

D

Danish, S., 37, 38, 43
D'Augelli, A., 32, 37, 38, 43
Davidson, E., 185, 197
Davidson, J., 180, 196
Davis, J., 23, 24, 25, 27, 43
Dean, J., 173, 196
Dohrenwend, B., 37, 38, 43
Dohrenwend, B.S., 37, 38, 43
Dorr, D., 38, 43
Drabman, R., 186, 196
Dworkin, A., 17, 43
Dworkin, E., 17, 43

E

Eisdorfer, C., 141
Eisenberg, J., 185, 197
Epperley, J., 160, 169

F

Farquhar, J., 186, 197
Field, J., 183, 196
Fine, M., 129, 136, 137, 141
Forrer, S., 160, 169
French, J., 118, 141

207

SUBJECT INDEX